Girlfriends'

❖ GUIDE TO ❖

WEIGHT
LOSS

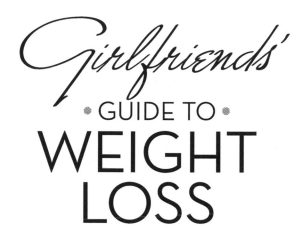

Girlfriends'
• GUIDE TO •
WEIGHT
LOSS

What Your Doctors Can't Tell You
and What Your Trainers Won't

IRENE GALLOS KOK

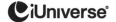

GIRLFRIENDS' GUIDE TO WEIGHT LOSS
WHAT YOUR DOCTORS CAN'T TELL YOU
AND WHAT YOUR TRAINERS WON'T

iUniverse books may be ordered through booksellers or by contacting:

iUniverse
1663 Liberty Drive
Bloomington, IN 47403
www.iuniverse.com
1-800-Authors (1-800-288-4677)

Because of the dynamic nature of the Internet, any web addresses or links contained in this book may have changed since publication and may no longer be valid. The views expressed in this work are solely those of the author and do not necessarily reflect the views of the publisher, and the publisher hereby disclaims any responsibility for them.

Any people depicted in stock imagery provided by Getty Images are models, and such images are being used for illustrative purposes only. Certain stock imagery © Getty Images.

ISBN: 978-1-5320-8175-0 (sc)
ISBN: 978-1-5320-8174-3 (e)

Library of Congress Control Number: 2019913078

Print information available on the last page.

iUniverse rev. date: 09/19/2019

I dedicate this book to my *parents* for
always loving and supporting me.
To my dad who showed me what hard work and
determination will bring with the proper mind-set.
To my mom for her strong will, passion for making
others happy, and amazing cooking skills.
I owe everything to their guidance.
Sorry I almost blew up the house cooking
that one time. Yes, that was me …

Acknowledgments

I cannot express enough thanks to my husband, Matt, for his continued support and encouragement. The endless hours of listening to me dictate sentences, offering assistance with word usage, and even doing household chores to make it possible to spend time writing. Thank you for always calling me beautiful and believing in me. I promise to stop ordering kitchen gadgets on Amazon so impulsively.

To my children who are my driving force. Seeing your smiling faces is the fuel in everything I do. I will always have memories of writing this book while cooking dinner and helping Sam and Aly with girl drama, all while the dogs were barking and Nic and Ava were arguing about something …

I wouldn't have it any other way. Special thanks to Alyssa for illustrating the cover of this book and adding extra life to the pages with her talented sketches. The book design was complete when she added Boston and Theo to the cover as they complete our NASA8 :)

To my brother who accompanied me in the kitchen as a young girl when my creativity began. Scalding hot chocolate pudding, sweet cream nacho cheese sauces, chunky guacamole, and mustard stains everywhere. I am not upset that you never got in trouble, as you have given me years of support and companionship and the perfect smile!

To my bestie, Kim, thank you for reading parts of this book as it evolved and encouraging me to continue writing it. Your encouragement when the times got rough is much appreciated and duly noted. I'm sorry for all those things I said when I was tired and crabby. That's what best friends are for ...

I sincerely appreciate the learning opportunities provided by my clients and friends. My completion of this project could not have been accomplished without the support of my work subjects. For those of you wondering if I would ever write a book about you, I finally did! Thank you for being my examples and for listening me talk endlessly about my book.

Introduction

For as long as I can remember, I have had two things on my bucket list: one was to run a marathon, and the other was to write a book. Clearly, the running thing was never going to happen, as back in my twenties, I couldn't run to the mailbox without having a stroke. Years ago, I decided I would write a book. I have started so many books over the past three decades that I can't even recall what they were even about. I decided that running a marathon might just be easier, and it was! In 2004 I ran my first marathon, and here I sit in from of my laptop with fifty marathon finishes fifteen years later and still no book.

Then I realized that I couldn't write a book because I didn't have a passion. I wasn't an expert in anything. As I sat and looked at the contact list of the thousands of clients with whom I have worked over the years, I realized that I am an expert.

I am not sure what makes me an expert. I can tell you that I am an expert of all the possible crap that anyone could come up with or encounter when trying to lose weight. Let me start out by saying that pretty much everything you read or see on the internet is a bunch of bullshit. Someone is trying to take your money. You see, money makes this world go 'round … and you are a target of a multigazillion-dollar industry. These industry peeps tell you pretty much anything to get you to click *order now*, and once you do … you're done. You have paid, and your hopes will be shattered. By the time you realize you have once again been fooled by the marketing giants of the world, it's too late.

I am not here to take your money. I am here to change your life. I am here to get you to see the real deal, as I have. It's not hard … but you have to dig deep. You have to get your feet wet and your hands dirty. You have to be patient and trust the process. The trust will get you here. Once you get here, it is the best place on earth. Many people have joined me on this journey, so lace up those shoes and let the rocky ride begin.

1

Get U Fit: Time to Get Real, Time to Get Fit

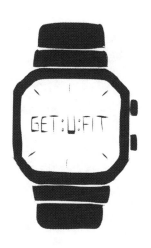

There is nothing that can get you ready for T-Day. Nothing. You wake up one day and decide you have had enough. This day is T-Day. T stands for *torture*. T-Day is the day you get to spend all day torturing about the pain and agony you feel. T-Day means you overamplify the ideas that you have let yourself go and embrace the reality of what a big fat cow you have become. You really are a fat cow. You eat like one. T-Day is the day are going to decide to get your ass in gear and do something about it. Since T-Day is the last day before you go on your lifelong trip to a wonderful new world, it is important that you mentally prepare for this new and challenging expedition.

Now please note … As a wellness coach, I dislike the word *fat*. It is demeaning, degrading, and disturbing. I never use that word unless I am describing a food's macronutrients. However, for this book, I will be using the word *fat* to make a dramatic impact, especially on a day like today, T-Day. So, let the torture begin. Whether you have five or one hundred pounds to lose, you need to say to yourself, "I have had enough of this garbage … I am tired of being a lazy sack of shit. I am good enough, I am strong enough, and I am going to like me!"

Are you ready?

Probably not.

Let's take it a step further.

Go to your closet right now.

Find your favorite pair of jeans that you know don't fit.

Put them on.

Go ahead … Put them on, even if they only get up to your knees.

For the love of God, look at yourself.

Is this torture enough?

We're not done …

Hobble yourself to the bathroom scale with those jeans wrapped around your ankles, and roll your fat ass on the scale. You heard me. Do it. Weigh yourself with the jeans on. I know you are thinking the jeans weigh a few pounds, but who fucking cares at this point. You obviously have a huge shit storm to clean up. You can brag about those extra pounds lost later.

It is time to face reality and admit to yourself what you weigh and then take a quick moment to think about how good you used to feel when you followed a plan. Think about how good you used to feel about having all that energy when you wanted to work out and looked forward to waking up early to go for a walk or run. Think of that mouthwatering desire to eat clean and healthy and how your metabolism flourished. Remember how you enjoyed exercise. Think about how you loved eating healthy foods and how you felt great about yourself. Not once did you think about how you looked because how you look becomes secondary to how you feel. Instead, you thought about how feeling better far outweighed looking better.

Take a moment to self-reflect …

What worked for you before?

What did you like best about that program?

How did you feel when you were succeeding in this plan?

At what point did you feel yourself slipping and why?

What would you do if you could do it again?

How will you incorporate what you have learned into this program?

Let's be real, people. We are the ones who have to walk around in our bodies all day long. Either we feel like a pile of dead weight crawling from under a rock, or we feel like we won the lottery and live on cloud nine. Why would anyone want to wake up tired and spend all day with stomach issues? Why would you want to be overweight; have high cholesterol, high blood pressure, and diabetes; go to bed tired; and live a life sentence of hell? For what? Crappy food that doesn't even taste good?

Don't get me wrong. That crappy food looks and smells good. The first bite may be okay … but after that, it's not good. I don't think anyone who has devoured a triple bacon cheeseburger and large serving of fries has ever felt *great* right after. Impossible. Yet, we continue to do it. We do it because we have become addicted to instant gratification. We do it because it is a habit. It is time to change those habits!

I will tell it what it is like to change those habits. I am here to tell you that I have been challenged like this many times. I can tell you what the jeans looked like. I can tell you what the scale said. I can also tell you that the last time I did this was the *last* time. I finally figured things out. I am using thirty years of personal experience along with twenty years of professional work to teach you how this process works and will be using actual stories from real clients. You will learn from all their mistakes. This process is not easy, so I will not sugarcoat the challenge. You need to learn and trust this process. And you need to trust me.

Before you get too excited about this, I should warn you. This is not your typical weight-loss book. It is not a book about calories, fat grams, or how to eat and exercise. While all of this is important, it comes secondary to what you will learn. This process is about learning the strategies to help you fight a mental battle with the proper tools and mind-set, as well as a positive outlook. You will learn to never surrender to your weaknesses and to keep your dreams alive. Weight loss will be a by-product of your new mind-set. In the following chapters, I will introduce you to some useful mental strategies to help you build a foundation for a new and challenging thought process. So let us get started!

2

Going Back to Kindergarten:
No Shortcuts

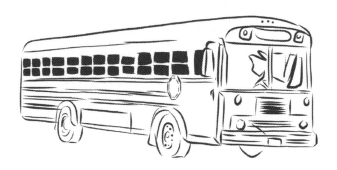

Since I am being realistic, you are not going to be ready for this life change in one day. You need to plan your start date at least a week in advance and ease into it. I never understood why people jump into such a drastic change in lifestyle overnight. This would be like moving to another country with no preparation whatsoever. If you knew you were moving to China, you would spend some time learning the language and studying the culture before moving there.

No wonder people get frustrated and quit. It is ridiculous to think someone who doesn't work out, meal prep, eat healthy, or drink water would start with a routine including all those things. Getting up early to make meals for the day, go workout for an hour, eat healthy foods all day, and know how to prepare everything doesn't happen overnight. What the fuck are you people thinking? That would be like me trying to put on scrubs, check into a hospital, and perform a surgical procedure on someone after watching one YouTube video. Let's be real. You need time. Like planning anything, you have to educate yourself and prepare yourself for the things that you will have to know and do. You should also note that it does not have to be done all at once.

Can you say the word *transition?* You could start slow and transition into more complex programs. Do not be that person I see at the checkout line at Walmart: the one with the food scale, bathroom scale, Vitamix, protein powder, chia seeds, almond milk, shaker bottles, meal prep containers, and hand weights all in their cart. Don't be a dumbass … Buying this shit isn't going to make you look good. There is more unused fitness equipment in the world than I would like to think about. Don't buy a damn thing yet. Let's start with throwing shit away and seeing what you already have at home.

You see, you only need real food and determination to make this work. Those gadgets are nice—trust me, I have them all—but I always use them. Once you get to that level, then you can invest in all this crap. Be forewarned. It takes up an ungodly amount of space in your house, and it will aggravate your spouse because you will keep ordering more.

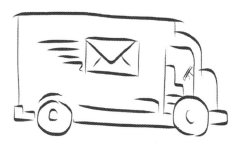

This is a touchy subject with my husband, but as everyone who knows me knows, I am the gadget queen. Thank goodness I work from home and can intercept the packages as they arrive daily. #primemember #lovemyhubby #heishot

So we agree; slow and steady wins the race. You are not starting tomorrow. We are still torturing ourselves. That part hasn't ended. Let's continue with those festivities …

In order for this to work, you need to set yourself up for success. You need to check what things you can change at first and what you feel you can change later. Let me give you an example. If you are someone who cannot get up early, do not fool yourself. Do not think you can suddenly pop out of bed like a lightning bolt. You will not be ready to work out like Jane Fonda with the sun shining and the birds chirping. *Wrong* … Do not do it. If you commit yourself to 5:00 a.m. workouts daily, you may end up only realistically doing this for a few weeks. You will end up disappointed early in the program.

Coffee is another example. Many of you start your day with this. It is the magic potion to people's sanity. If you are a cream-and-sugar kind of gal and you cannot drink it otherwise, then this should be something you keep at first.

Now reeeeelaxxxxxx … I am not saying to keep all your favorite things, just the ones you know you will need at first. Keep in mind that your progress may be delayed a bit depending on the habits you are unwilling to change. The time will pass either way, and slow and steady wins the race … *right?!*

Okay, now that we have that done … We have to make our list of things we have to change. Let's analyze this word. *Change*. By definition, the verb *change* means "to make or become different; to alter, adjust, revamp, transform, redesign and reorganize." That is exactly what I want you to do.

Change

[cheynj]

Verb (used with object) [changed. Change‣ing]

1. to make the form, nature, content, future course, etc. of (something) different from what it is or from what it would be if left alone; to change one's name; to change one's opinion; to change the course of history

2. to transform, reorganize, adjust, alter, or convert (usually followed by into): The witch changed the prince into a toad.

3. to substitute another or others for; exchange for something else, usually of the same kind: She changed her shoes when she got home from the office.

By definition, the verb *change* means "to make or become different; to alter, adjust, revamp, transform, redesign and reorganize."

That is exactly what I want you to do.

Reorganize, Adjust, Alter Redesign, Transform

There is no way you can expect yourself to make such extreme changes to the way you eat and live 24/7. Let's put this into perspective. Let's pretend you are starting kindergarten. You are going to school to learn the basics. You will learn how to color, draw, write your name, add, and subtract. You will not worry about learning how to multiply and divide until you are ready. It amazes me how people who have a lot of weight to lose worry about the percentages of protein and carbohydrates in the food they are eating.

Although the percentages of protein and carbohydrates are something of importance, you should not worry about them during the first week, or even month, on a diet. It isn't relevant if you're overloaded with information that your brain can't compute. This is how people get overwhelmed and end up eating a burger. They get fluckstrated* and quit.

Fluckstrated

[fluks-trey-tid]

(adjective)

1. disappointed past the normal level of being frustrated; an amplified version of frustration; thwarted: The mom was fluckstrated that her child would not stop screaming.
2. having a feeling of or filled with fluckstration; dissatisfied: His unresolved difficulty left him absolutely fluckstrated.

You're in frickin' kindergarten.

Stop trying to dissect a frog.

Save that for middle school.

You are not hiring a demolition team to knock down your house and build a new one. You are updating the one you live in. Make alterations as you can tolerate, and continue to make extra adjustments as you evolve with the program.

Ground Rules

Since we're going back to school, let's lay down some ground rules. There will be no cutting in line, no cheating, and no copying off your neighbor's test for answers. I have cut in line so many times when trying to lose weight. If there was a jail for line cutters, I would have a life sentence without parole. While I agree that the quick-and-easy way seems the most appealing, the quick-and-easy way will get you nowhere in life and will definitely get you nowhere in a weight-management program. I am going to take a moment to define each of these violations.

Cutting in Line

Our society is always looking for shortcuts. People pay big bucks to have things expedited and shipped overnight. We are used to this premier service, in which you pay extra and can cut in line. Simple … The faster the better. Right? Amazon ships overnight. Supermarkets deliver groceries to your door in two hours. Even Uber will bring you a Big Mac and large fries on demand with the flash of an Apple Pay. This is our culture.

In the eighties, we had microwaves to cook a TV dinner in three minutes, not in the forty-five minutes that the oven used to take. Now we have Instant Pots that can make pot roast in twenty-five minutes instead of in four hours. Fast … faster … faster.

When you are in kindergarten and the teacher says you can have a sip of water, you have two choices: patiently wait your turn or cut in line. If you wait your turn, then you get to enjoy your three sips of water. You can savor every bit of the crisp, refreshing moment as you take your three sips. If you cut in line, you may get to the water faster, but you run the risk of getting caught and having to go back to the end of the line, humiliated and embarrassed. What happens when you cut in line? You may get ahead for a short moment, but then you end up going way back to where you started.

How do you cut in line with weight loss?

Let's see … This could be a book in itself.

Quick fixes: pills, cleanses, and detoxes, along with all the other bullcrap you see on TV that makes you want to lose a hundred pounds in ten days. You will lose weight by taking diet pills, which will curb your appetite, and you will not be hungry. You will also lose weight if you drink lemon juice mixed with distilled water and maple syrup for fifteen straight days with no food.

Newsflash: You will lose weight if you drink shakes all day and have a sensible dinner.

Sensible dinner, my ass …

Whoever came up with that line must not have choked on a bone while inhaling the entire fucking chicken because they were starving.

Just saying.

Yet we all know that kind of hunger after drinking shakes all day.

Let's stop and take a quick trip down memory lane. Do the words *eat your arm off* hit the spot? If you're nodding your head, then you're being honest. This is what happens to your system when you are hungry.

If you let yourself get really hungry, you are screwed.

Not just a little screwed but the kind of screwed where you want to rewind but can't. The self-pity, why-did-I-do-this, I-am-so-mad, Goddamn-it, I-was-doing-so-good kind of screwed.

You're nodding your head again?

Yep …

You see, it's not all your fault.

Pay close attention to this because it will change the way you perceive hunger. There are certain things you cannot control, and how your body works is one of them. Food and nutrition are basic needs for survival. Our bodies will tell us to eat in order to survive. Our systems will fight if we try to mess with our natural instincts. My advice to you is don't mess with it. When we are hungry and ready for food and nourishment, our brains send signals to alert us that we need to eat. Smelling food will cause salivation to occur. As soon as we start salivating, our bodies' digestive enzymes in our stomachs will begin secreting enzymes to help digest food once we do eat. In the meantime, the enzymes are also sending more signals to our brains to eat. If we don't eat, the urge to eat becomes more and more intense and will not subside until we nourish our bodies. The longer we wait, the more illogical we become.

Don't laugh. This is true. Think about it. When you get to this point of stupid hungry, you don't care about calories or your food plan. You need to eat. The hunger isn't in your control, which isn't even the worse part. The worst part is that whatever you decide to taste first is going to be your demise for the night. Dare to put a potato chip in your mouth during this hunger phase, and you will eat the entire bag in moments. Care for a small bite of cheese to tide you over while you make dinner? Sure … one the size of Wisconsin.

You know I speak the truth here.

The bottom line is you cannot allow yourself to get to this point of hunger. If you do, your body's natural tendencies will take over. Evil little monsters who live in the depths of your brain are slowly woken by the sounds of your grumbling tummy. These monsters cause you to make illogical food choices that you will later regret. You probably aren't aware of these little fuckers, as no doctor will ever warn you about them. No worries … We will meet them later in this book, as I don't want to scare you away so soon … But for now, follow my lead.

Cheating

Cheating is for cheaters. Don't be a cheater. Cheaters often get ahead for a short time but undoubtedly finish last. Sometimes they don't even finish. They become cheaters who do not finish. Athletes who cheat have their gold metals stripped for performance-enhancing drug use. Judges have been pulled off benches for fixed elections. Millionaires have gone to prison for white-collar crimes that made them rich.

Gamblers have been caught on video hiding cards. Women have caught their husbands cheating over many centuries. Every one of these people were living the high life at one point, thinking all of their dreams had come true. Unfortunately, they took a huge cut in line. The front-cut kind that Susie Koepenkegger always took on the way to gym class year after year, until the one year when she got caught. Susie tripped and fell down the stairs and couldn't go on the end of the year field trip to the zoo. #notworthit #susiewasstupid

Diet cheaters are no different. Keep in mind that I am not talking about *cheating on your diet*. I am talking about being a *diet cheater*. There is a difference. Someone who is a diet cheater is someone who is trying to get ahead by taking shortcuts and not following the rules. This is very common with weight loss. Everyone wants the fastest way to shed unwanted fat. Cutting your calories low will drop your weight fast. Once you get into the groove, you may find that skipping meals and snacks isn't so bad. As you see numbers on the scale drop, so does your desire to ever snack again. The next thing you know, you may find yourself getting eight hundred calories a day and dropping three pounds a week. During this time, you will actually feel good. Your body will adapt to this caloric deficit. The euphoric high you feel from shedding the weight will carry you through the desire to splurge. Some people can maintain this for weeks, some for months, and others can continue this for years. The reality is that no one can sustain it forever.

The day will come when your body will decide it needs more nourishment. This process is gradual. Usually, it starts with a small increase in calories. First you will add snacks back or other foods that you eliminated. Initially, the scale won't move up because your body is still confused. So then you inevitably increase your intake even more. I call this the honeymoon stage in weight loss. It's great until the honeymoon is over. Suddenly, you come home to the reality of a snoring husband, credit card bills, and an annoying mother-in-law. Oops … Sorry, that happened in my first marriage. #badjoke #couldnthelpit

Once the honeymoon is over, you will then see the numbers on the scale creep up, but this time, you will see the number creep up in a different way. Because you deprived your body of nourishment for an extended period of time and then replenished it with a surplus of calories all at once, your body is going to hold on to this new surplus of calories for dear life in fear of the deprivation you gave it. To top it off, you now feel defeated, bloated, and disgusted. You have no energy.

I know, I know, you feel the pain. It doesn't end here. This cheater decides she is going to go back to her brilliant eight-hundred-calorie-a-day plan again after the weekend because it worked before. She has one last feeding fest and stuffs her face like she is going to be hibernating for the winter. Monday comes and goes, and after months of this battle, this cheater is standing in the back of the line once again.

It doesn't pay. Stick to the plan, let your body lose weight as it finds appropriate, and you won't end up with a messed-up metabolism and a shattered ego. If the plan is not healthy and realistic, then it is not the plan for you.

Over-Exercising

Another way people try to take shortcuts with a weight-loss process is by overdoing their activity levels. Stop everything before you continue. Look at the last sentence in the last paragraph above: *If it is not healthy and realistic—* healthy and realistic—Your activity levels should be healthy and realistic.

First of all, you will never meet anyone who enjoys working out as much as me. Was I always like this? Hell no. I was the one who hated exercise, but now that I am transformed, it is part of my everyday life. As I have been getting older, I am needing to have it. The arthritis sets in at a certain age, and you will find yourself exercising for reasons that do not include getting a six-pack. Whatever you decide as your plan, it should be realistic. As mentioned earlier, start slowly. If you are not currently working out, then incorporating some walks a few days a week is a great start.

Walking is underrated. I love to walk and actually believe that walking has been the secret to how I have been able to maintain my weight over the years. What am I saying? I am implying that no matter what your level is, incorporating walking into your routine is very realistic. Be realistic. Start planning how you can add little walks or workouts into your day without having to restructure your entire schedule. If you can walk during lunch, start incorporating that into your day. If you can get to the office a little early and do some cardio in the fitness center, that could be a realistic plan as well. Even doing a YouTube yoga class during a break on occasion could add variety to your routine.

Proceed with caution because sometimes you may not even realize that you are traveling to Cheater's Town. You may truly enjoy your routine. For example, suppose you are a runner and have the kind of job where you can go running every day at lunch. In making the decision to do this, you find that you enjoy it and are able to fit it in. You tell yourself you can do this. Yet, be warned. This has *cheater* written all over it. Are you confused? So was Cassandra. Allow me to share her story.

> Cassandra started losing weight last year and had a hard time fitting in exercise. She used to be a runner. Now as a fifth-grade teacher and mother of two small children, she doesn't have the time. One day, she decided to go for a walk during her forty-five-minute lunch break. This felt great. The next day she packed her running gear and went for a quick run. Oh my goodness, this was the best day ever! Cassandra hit the jackpot here. She could plug in her music and get her run in every single day without

trying to figure out when she could fit in exercise.

Cassandra had her system down to a perfect science. The bell rang, and she ran to the bathroom and changed into her running clothes. She would dart out the door and run three miles every day during her lunch hour. She would rush back, race through the halls as she wiped the sweat off, and change back into her teacher clothes. All this in time for her twenty-four students to come busting through the door, ready for her to calm them down for math. She did it, yet it wasn't always easy.

Some days, she would have to cut someone short on a conversation so she could make it out the door. Other times, she was unable to regroup or recollect her thoughts from a stressful morning. Many times, she excluded herself from social lunch outings with the other teachers to go running. There was also the stress of getting back to school on time. Once, she got lost, which caused her to get back a few minutes late in sweaty running clothes. Another time, she lost her earbuds on a run and had to retrace her steps later to find them. The worst was when she needed to use the bathroom during a run and ended up wasting the entire forty-five minutes getting to a gas station. She had to sprint back to get ten minutes of exercise in with no time to eat her lunch. She was starting to dislike her afternoon run sessions but didn't want to admit it to herself yet. She was only missing lunch.

Oh … Yes, lunch, or in Cassandra's case it was no lunch. Cassandra would skip eating lunch (super cheater in progress). Run and skip lunch. She looked great, of course, and she had a front-row spot in the Happy Parade. She looked healthy and felt healthy. Although she was skipping lunch, she would drink a protein shake at her desk as her students worked on their math problems. She was getting her calories in but not eating lunch—you know, the food kind that you chew at a table with your friends, while you talk and take a break from the hectic day. Cassandra dropped weight faster than a tree drops its leaves in the fall, but she would suffer the long-term consequences for this cheating behavior.

The weather changed. Cassandra did not run on school holidays or on days when her own kids were home sick. Cassandra got tired of packing and unpacking sweaty clothes every day. Now that it was cold, she needed to pack heavier gear, and more of it. It took twice as long to put on this cold running gear and thrice as long to take it off.

When she did run, she would not enjoy it as much in the cold, wind, rain, and ice. Many days she would skip it. Not knowing if she was going to skip her run, she would still pack all her gear up and only bring her protein shake for lunch. After a while, she got tired of drinking her shake and felt uncomfortable going to the teachers' lounge. She hadn't been there in months, so she would drive some place to get a quick bite and bring it back or eat lunch in her car. Although Cassandra was well liked, she felt unwelcome at lunch. Others were starting to make comments such as, "Gee, Cassandra, why aren't you running anymore?" Or, "We knew you couldn't maintain this running thing forever." Once, she actually heard one of the older teachers say, "I could have told her she wasn't going to be able to keep that up." Cassandra eventually stopped running during her lunch hour and gained back most of her weight within a few months.

How could this have happened so quickly? There were several factors that contributed to Cassandra's weight gain. Here is a simple breakdown:

- ✦ Cassandra lost her gusto and did not want to run during lunch anymore. With an average calorie burn of 400 calories each day from running, this equaled a 2,000-calorie difference in a week (400 x 5 = 2,000).
- ✦ Cassandra began eating an average lunch instead of her shake. This equaled a 1,500- to 2,000-calorie surplus a week. Her shake was 300 calories. Her unplanned lunches totaled an average of 800 calories a day: a 500-calorie surplus (500 x 5 = 2,500 each week).

Due to the circumstances, Cassandra had the potential to gain 1.2 pounds each week. This weight gain led to a very bruised ego and a complete derailment. Once she was unable to run, she stopped exercising altogether. She gained back most of her weight. She didn't need to, but her inability to stay on this unrealistic routine was the demise of her eating program as well.

You may ask, "Am I not allowed to work out during my lunch?" It may work for some people but not for everyone; and in this case, it was not realistic. If it is realistic for you, then it could definitely work. Perhaps you work from home and do not need to rush to change into workout apparel.

Or you could eat an actual lunch while on a conference call. Maybe you could get on a treadmill on cold days. You might have a facility at your office with showers, making it easier to transition back to work. In these cases, exercising at work may be a possibility.

There is a fine line to what makes a person an exercise cheater, but many people are guilty of it. Here are some other common exercise cheater violations:

+ Working out multiple times a day
+ Packing weights and exercise bands so you can exercise on the go
+ Waking up at three o'clock in the morning to exercise and then not being able to function for the rest of the day
+ Leaving your kids at the sitter longer every night to work out
+ Trying to burn more calories than you eat

These exercise behaviors may be fine for those who can sustain these habits. You need to ask yourself if what you are doing is realistic before doing it every day. Otherwise, you will regret it.

Copying Off Your Neighbor's Paper

This kind of cheating is also very dangerous. Like in school, the temptation of getting the answers from the smart kid in class is so great. You're overtaken by a small glance at his paper just to see what he is doing. It is human nature to have self-doubt. It is normal to want to know what someone else is doing, especially if it is working for that other person. The problem with getting answers from someone else is that you are not doing the actual work. You will never learn what you are intended to. If a food plan asks you to log calories and you look up approximate values of similar foods instead, this may cost you later. Your program may need you to learn how to food prep and create grocery lists. If you get these lists from friends, you will never build the habits needed to make this part of your regular routine. You are wrong again if you think that what your neighbor is eating will work for you. You will not miraculously fit into her size-2 designer jeans by copying her grocery list.

Do you want to see me lose my shit?

Someone comes up to me at a party and asks me to tell them exactly what I eat and how I exercise. Apparently, people think they can repeat my routine just like that. They want to skip the thirty years of blood, sweat, and tears that it took to finally fit into my overpriced jeans. They forget about the work it takes to make sure my ass doesn't ever bust out of them.

Stop thinking that you can do what other people do.

It will not work for you the same way.

We are a box of crayons.

We may all look similar, but everything about our insides is different.

In the grand scheme of things, we are the same. There are way too many variables for anyone to think she can copy someone else's exact regime and have it work. As you start shining like a super star and your friends all want to copy off your homework, be sure you explain this process with extreme caution. The most critical variable of all is the level of determination that you may have going into the program. If you are not motivated, repeating the exact same program that once worked for you may not work a second time. Crayons … Remember, same but different. Things may have changed, one of which may be your attitude and level of determination. Think about that long and hard before you continue, and *please* keep your eyes on your own damn paper.

in a treadmill or heart rate monitor. Educate yourself and make those purchases. Any psychiatrist could tell you that people use shopping as a form of therapy. In this case, buying fitness equipment that you will never use may serve as a form of self-torture.

There are a few things that I find necessary to help guide success in the right direction. You need an accurate bathroom scale, kitchen scale, measuring cups and spoons, and method of food logging and calculation. I am not saying you can't be successful without these items. These tools are critical in the mind-set and motivation needed to be successful in a weight-management program. I have had many people, both qualified and not, try to argue with me about this point. It boils down to a matter of opinion and what works for each individual. If you want to be a true badass, get yourself a decent bathroom scale, kitchen scale, and measuring tools. I have had the pleasure of working with all types of people. I am going to provide the appropriate criteria to avoid confusion. The last time I didn't clarify what type of kitchen scale to buy, someone was using an old US mail scale that he bought at a garage sale. That person ended up gaining weight because his two-dollar deal was giving him inaccurate measurements.

Choosing a Bathroom Scale

Stop everything right now!

Right frickin' now …

If you listen to anything I tell you to do, this is one that ranks high on the list.

Do not …

I repeat …

Do not buy a cheap bathroom scale here.

If you are going to try to save a penny on anything, save it elsewhere. I cannot believe how many people minimize the importance of investing in a valid and accurate scale. We are not talking about spending a million dollars here. We are talking about spending the difference between a twenty-dollar scale and a fifty-dollar scale. For the love of God … the extra thirty dollars will be worth the countless hours of doubt you will have if your old bathroom scale does not work.

You are going to spend twenty-four hours every single day, seven days every single week working as hard as you possibly can. You will wake up every day with the hope of seeing the number on the scale go down. But your 1902 Woolworth Model Q52 scale won't budge if it is older than shit. You will want to pay someone more than thirty dollars to lock your crazy ass in a padded room for the day. Need I say more?

Don't get all happy-in-the-pants excited to throw away your old bathroom scale yet. First, let's be sure it is ready for retirement. We know you want to get rid of it because we know that scale is completely at fault for you not being able to lose any weight over the last ten years. To be fair, we should run the proper diagnostics on it to be sure. This test will most likely need to be done to any of your scales in the future to ensure their accuracy. You may want to highlight this section for future use.

Testing Your Scale for Accuracy and Validity

1. Get on and off of it five times. The weight should be within a few ounces for all five assessments. If the scale gives you five completely different weights, it is a piece of shit and needs to be thrown away immediately. No further testing required. It is time to buy a new one.

2. If your scale passed step 1, you should get on the scale holding a ten-pound weight. The scale should say you weigh exactly ten pounds more. Repeat

this test three more times. You should get the same weight within a few ounces to continue on to step 3. If your scale does not say you weigh ten pounds more, then then we have a problem … *pitch* …

3. The true test is in your being able to manipulate your scale and not interfere with the accuracy of it. Get on your scale in a variety of different ways: sideways, tiptoes, standing in the middle, standing on the end. A good scale will give you the same number whether you are standing on your head or holding your breath. You should weigh the same. That's right folks. We have all done this. Getting a good scale will save you hours of fucking around in the bathroom, trying to see the number drop a measly ounce as if it matters because it actually does.

If you work hard, you should get to see the result. If you screw up and devour an entire deep-dish pizza and sleeve of Oreos, then you want that bastard of a scale to look at you in the face and say it like it is. The Model Q52 would most likely have no clue of the damage done; therefore, neither would you. You will be getting on this fucker 365 times a year, and that is assuming you only weigh once a day. In one year alone, a one-hundred-dollar scale costs you three cents a day. Please keep in mind that I will stress we are not doing this just for weight loss. The bottom line is we are driven by the number on the scale, and we shouldn't be misguided … #dontbeacheapass

Kitchen Measuring Tools

As much as you would like to think you know how much a tablespoon or an ounce is, chances are that you are miscalculating. Underestimating the amount of lettuce you put on your tuna sandwich will have no impact on your weight loss. On the other hand, miscalculating the amount of salad dressing you put on your salad day after day will add up. Something as calorically dense as oil or peanut butter can be spread out and add will up pretty quickly.

Here's a newsflash: a standard kitchen spoon is not necessarily one tablespoon in mass. My fancy-dancy Pottery Barn stemware includes spoons that are more like little fishbowls. I was loving my celery sticks with two tablespoons peanut butter twice a day. I should have known I was eating way more than two tablespoons of peanut butter because I was busting out of my yoga pants. The peanut butter jar said it contained thirty-two servings, which should have taken me way longer to eat than the three days it took me to suck down the entire jar. This should have been the writing on the wall. You see, I didn't want to look at that writing on the wall. I was too busy inhaling the peanut butter like it was my last meal, squeezed into my skin-tight lululemons.

I was pretending that it was two tablespoons and only 210 calories. After all, it was healthy, all-natural, organic peanut butter with added omega-3s and flaxseeds.

Did I say inhaling?

Okay … I lied. I stuck my face in the jar and made sure I got every last bite of the 210-calorie serving treat out. After all … The more I could fit on my spoon, the better, right?

Ha!

Guilty, right?

It's okay … I told you I wouldn't call bullshit in this book. I have done it, and you have done it.

I was ignoring and miscalculating the amount of peanut butter I was eating. Until I came to terms with this, I could never free myself from blaming my lack of weight loss on hormones or a malfunctioning thyroid.

It's simple. I was kidding myself. The real truth was that I did not really want to measure the peanut butter because if

I did, I knew that I would be getting a lot less peanut butter than I was used to getting. I said that wrong. It's going to be a lot less peanut butter—so much less that you will actually question the impracticality of measuring peanut butter.

What is worse is that when you do eat the measly tablespoon of peanut butter, you will be appalled that such a small amount could be so high in calories. For God's sake, you don't even get enough peanut butter to spread across the celery stick. You will then find yourself licking the spoon so clean that it will shine like you polished it with a jewelry cloth. Furthermore, you will never have celery and peanut butter as a snack again.

This is one example—just one. So get yourself some measuring cups and spoons, along with a kitchen scale. If you ever question why you cannot lose weight on a food plan or why diets never work for you, it is because you are not measuring. Even after decades of using measuring tools, I still find myself miscalculating, which could lead to either weight gain or feelings of failure. Don't waste your time doing everything right but then doing everything wrong. Measure the goddamn peanut butter, assuming you ever eat it again.

A Food Log or Journal

First off, put the credit card down. This isn't something you get to go out and buy. It could be notebook or journal. You can be 2019 and use an app instead of going with the Thomas Jefferson version of logging it in a journal, which can simply be in the form of a notebook. Decide which method you want to use and become familiar with it. If you are going to use an app, then do some online research for reviews on well-known, user-friendly food-logging apps. Select one that has a large database with many users. Don't go cheap here. You'll regret it.

If you are old-school and want to actually log your food the good old-fashioned written way, that works as well. As a lifelong food logger, I can recall my fondest memories of breaking out my felt-tip markers to color code my meals. I would draw huge arrows and smiley faces when I met a weight-loss goal. Those were the days, although I do enjoy getting a digital fireworks display on my phone when I drink all my water. Once I got so obsessed that I went with a 1902 calligraphy pen and a 2017 modern app world at the same time. I felt like I was on top of the world logging in my journal and on my iPhone all at once. It was like My Fitness Pal meets Richard Simmons. Then I concluded and realized how ridiculous I was. I needed to get a journal that had a pocket for my iPhone to make things easier. That has nothing to do with this book, so I'll talk about my silly inventions later. I may have an entire catalog of things by the time I'm done writing this book. Save your money for then. You're not shopping for now.

Once you have chosen your method of food logging, start recording what you eat and developing a habit of writing down every morsel and bite that goes into your mouth. Lucky for you, we will discuss this further later in this book when we start getting serious.

4

Making This the Last First Day of Your Diet

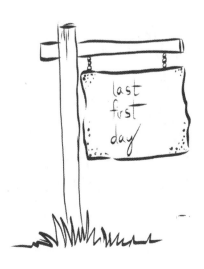

One thing that has always intrigued me is why people always feel compelled to have a start date and end date. I find this ridiculous! If you are starting something and plan on ending it, then you really have no plan to stay on or maintain the program. When I book a vacation, I have a start and end date for my trip. I plan on going to my destination, staying there, and enjoying the culture while I am there. Then I plan on returning home to my regular routine by the end date.

Why does a health and wellness program have to be so cut and dry? Is this how we are wired—with deadlines and due dates? No, not when you consider your health and wellness. You need to go into this with the understanding that this program is permanent—something that you plan for the long term. Before you begin this program, or any program, think of the changes you will make as a true lifelong commitment and include the modifications needed to make this plan realistic and sustainable.

This of this first day of your diet. It will be just like any other day in your crazy life. Do not set it up as if it were a special day. People always start their diets on a special day. They include special ceremonies and traditions that will be replayed over and over on those first days every single time they start a diet, over and over, again and again. Enough already! For you, this first day will be the very last first day of a diet that you will ever experience. Treat this day as if it were any normal day. Do not glorify it. Do not brag about it. Do not be nervous. Do not lose sleep over it. This is it—the first day of the rest of your life. Go easy and go into this program with that mind-set.

You have to change some things but do not have to be too drastic. You will not be able to sustain the change if you make too many overwhelming changes. For example, no one in in his or her right mind initially thinks raw broccoli and raw onion taste good. Eventually, they will taste so frickin' good that you will crave that broccoli, onion, bacon, cheese, and mayo salad. Your taste buds will be cultured, and you will enjoy even the most pungent flavors. Broccoli and onion will eventually taste good!

By the way, the broccoli and onion are only put in this signature dish so dumbasses like you think they're eating something healthy. You're actually fooling yourself. Look up the calories on this salad, and you will go back to eating your peanut butter.

Whether acquired or inborn, we can become accustomed to certain food flavors. We need to open our minds. I am going to give you some important advice, which will change your ability to manage your weight for the rest of your life

Golden Girlfriend Survival Rule 1

Eat to fuel your body.

Do not eat exclusively for pleasure.

Let your body decide which foods are best.

Do not let your mind chose which foods are best.

Take a minute to read that and break it down.

Read between the lines.

Eat to Fuel Your Body

In primitive years, the cave people ate to survive. It did not matter what they ate or how they ate it: cold, hot, cooked, or raw. It did not matter. They also determined which foods gave them energy, which foods made them lethargic, and which foods to avoid. They did not read diet books or nutritional labels. Cave people ate exactly what they needed for their bodies. There were few if no overweight people, and they saw fewer cases of health-related diseases, high blood pressure, high cholesterol, and diabetes. Certain cancers were nonexistent.

Do you think they ate for pleasure? We cannot answer that question. I am sure they had the chance to select foods they enjoyed over foods they did not like. Guess what? So will you—as long as you always remember that you are eating to fuel your body. Eating is not a sport or a hobby or an event.

The primary purpose of eating food is to provide energy and nutrition for your body, and you will need enough fuel to get yourself through several hours of living until it is time to refuel again. The fuel you select can be one that you enjoy, but the main purpose of eating is for the nutrients that the food provides. The main purpose of eating is not only to chew, taste, and overindulge. You will be chewing, tasting, and enjoying the food as you consume it. Although you should enjoy the food you consume, eating should not be your favorite pastime.

If we exercised Golden Girlfriend Survivor Rule 1 more often, there would be no other rules. There would be no other chapters in this book. I would be able to plop on the couch and write a book about something else. Instead, I have to spend God knows how much longer writing the rest of this book, so you morons can get this shit right. So please start considering food as fuel and not entertainment. You have had enough fun. Time to get serious.

Next, you need to think about how eating certain foods puts you in a danger zone. We all have these so-called foods, trigger foods, or foods that put us in the danger zone. These foods put us at risk for a total diet disaster. You may think these foods are healthy in nature, but when you so much as look at them, you tend to fall off your diet.

It took me years to realize that these evil monsters even existed. For example, I knew I loved guacamole a lot. If I was at a party, I would eat a lot of it and ruin my appetite by eating so much of it. This is all information I knew, party after party, year after year, and derailment after derailment. Why did it take me more than twenty years to figure out that guacamole was a danger-zone food? Whenever there was guacamole at a party, I just wanted to dive into the bowl and swim in the creamy green glob, all while taking mouthfuls. However, I determined that If I avoided the guacamole, I could get through the party without compromising whatever success I had achieved on my diet. What I started to do was to plan better. I would simply plan *not* to eat my danger-zone foods because once I did, my taste buds were triggered and wanted to only eat that food.

Never choose to start a meal with a danger-zone food. You will basically be programming your taste buds to want an endless amount of that food. Your brain is not capable of stopping your hands from shoveling that danger-zone food into your chewing mouth, whether the danger-zone food be guacamole, bean dip, popcorn, cheese, french fries, ice cream, oatmeal, or bridge mix. You should identify what foods you need to stay away from and step away from them immediately.

Jump into the guacamole bowl, my friends. Enjoy your swim and don't choke on an avocado chunk.

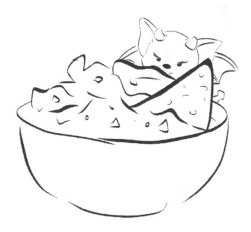

Notice I didn't say *avoid*; I said step away. Think about it. Evaluate it. Plan and decide if you should have it. Decide how much you should have. Think about your thinking. Do not get sucked over to the danger-zone food like a robot and start shoveling the food into your mouth.

Golden Girlfriend Survival Rule 2

Identify your danger zone foods.

Never eat them first.

Think about your thinking.

Always plan wisely.

Stop it right now!

The first day, and two rules learned. You have not purchased anything. I have saved you hundreds of dollars. You have already saved yourself thousands of calories by practicing what I have taught you. Can you imagine how much you will love me in another hundred pages?! I can't even stand it.

The next two rules are extremely important, but unfortunately, these two rules are not as simple. If this process was a simple one, it would be a beautiful world—a world where calories didn't count and jeans never got tight. In reality, our metabolism slows down as we age. Our boobs get sagier with each child we bear. These things happen. We can't stop it, so we just have to face it ... which brings me to my next rule.

Golden Girlfriend Survival Rule 3

Stop lying to yourself.

I cannot believe the extreme state of denial that people put themselves in when it comes to losing weight. It is downright insane what some people have convinced themselves of. If you are sitting there thinking, *not me*, then wake up from this state of denial that you have been in for all these years. On this very last first day of your diet, you need to stop sugarcoating shit and start seeing things as they are. I cannot believe the outrageous level of denial that people put themselves in when it comes to losing weight. It is downright insane what people have convinced themselves of over the years.

Repeat after me: "I am a dumbass if I have not fooled myself into convincing myself about something that I have wanted to believe. I am an even bigger idiot for thinking I could get away with it."

Now that you have declared that, what exactly have you been lying to yourself about? You believe something is wrong with you, your metabolism, your thyroid, your hormones. You may think you are pregnant or that you have a stomach tumor.

If I could make you feel better, allow me to list some of the more common fallacies that you may be honoring at the moment that need to be put to rest. These are the primary reasons why you haven't been able to succeed in a weight loss plan—the main reasons why you believe there is something wrong with you. It is not your metabolism, your thyroid, or your hormones. You are not pregnant. You do not have a stomach tumor. You do not have anything wrong with you that would cause you not to lose weight. You are not the only person on earth with the most fucked up metabolism ever known to man.

Please don't get these confused with excuses. Excuses are a far different and more complicated subject that I will cover much later in this book. Lies are fables or stories that you have told. In this case, you have told them to yourself so often that you have started to believe them. You have now convinced yourself these reasons are true. You have fallen into the category of fat-ass dumbass. Once again, I will apologize for the political incorrectness of my terminology. As I stated earlier, you're only a fat-ass and a dumbass when you love yourself enough to admit you aren't perfect. Whether you have one pound to lose or ninety-nine, you are reading this book to create better wellness habits. One of them is admitting that you are some form of an ass. I am an ass. My husband is an ass. It doesn't have to be a bad thing. That, and I was mad at him the other day for something stupid. #istilllovehim #hesthebest #dontlietoyourself #pantsonfire

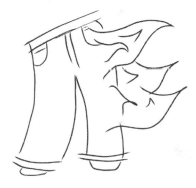

What follows are some of the more common reasons people use to blame for their inability to lose weight. As you read them over, think about each one and how it relates to you. Think about whether you have used any of these reasons as an excuse for not being able to succeed on a plan. For now, how you will now go into this new way of life with a different mind-set?

"All those little bites of food don't add up to much."

Really, people? Weight Watchers came up with the BLTs (bites, licks, and tastes). Even though we all know that everything we put in our mouths counts as calories, we still refuse to count them as calories. A grape, a piece of sugar-free gum, a sip of soda, a bite of a donut ... Let's be real. These BLTs add up to hundreds and even thousands of calories. One time I was up ten pounds and couldn't figure out why. I was dumbfounded. I knew what I was doing but couldn't imagine that my grazing could do such damage. Between the almonds, gummy bears, gum, peanut butter licks, sips of soda, unmeasured salad dressing, random grapes, and goldfish crackers, I had a nice muffin top to show for it. Don't laugh. This is a true story. I really did measure my bites one day: 878 calories later, I decided to sew my mouth shut the next day.

"I'm gaining weight, but it's because I am building muscle."

The last person who came to me with this theory ended up losing forty-five pounds after I reprogrammed her brain. I taught her the basics of weight loss. She was bullshitting herself. When you catch yourself thinking the scale has gone up because you have gained muscle, go back and reread that last sentence to yourself. Do it in front of the mirror. No one has ever lost weight on a program and ended up weighing more than when they began.

Muscle does weigh more than fat; in fact, muscle weighs a lot more. If you started a food plan weighing 187 pounds; ate a high-protein, low-carb diet; and then weighed 195 pounds a few weeks later, you may have gained some muscle, but you should have also lost some body fat. Further, if you were lifting weights at the gym, your frame should have gotten smaller. Again, don't lie to yourself. Look at what you are doing. Furthermore, fat does not turn into muscle. They are two completely different forms of human tissue. One does not turn into the other.

"I'm not eating enough calories, so that's why I'm not losing weight."

Dear Lord. Those of you who know me can see my eyes rolling back and me biting my lip right now. We can thank the weight-loss reality shows for this brain fuck. All right, here's how it goes … If you don't get enough calories, you will lose weight. You will not go into starvation mode after three or four days or even three or four weeks, for the love of God.

Starvation mode is a true thing. When you have dozens (and even hundreds) of pounds to lose, your body is going to burn that fat like an inferno. As soon as you don't provide fuel to your body, it has to use your body fat as energy. Let's think about this. Have you ever seen a weight-loss reality show contestant *not* lose weight? Do you know why? It is because they are actually following the program. All of the contestants have an overabundance of body fat, and during the show, they are using their excess body fat for their bodies' energy.

None of those people are getting enough calories. None of them. They are all put in unrealistic scenarios where they are given 1,200 to 1,400 calories a day to feed their two-hundred-plus-pound bodies. Then are told to exercise twelve or more hours a day. That is not enough calories. They lose weight, and they do it under unrealistic measures for the television viewers to watch and for ratings to go up.

Even though those people are not getting enough calories, starvation mode for them has not really kicked in. In reality, the body does not starve until the body is at the point of survival. If you have an overabundance of body fat, your body will use it for energy. It will not starve.

As far as those reality show contestants, most of them do end up gaining the weight back due to the extreme measures that were taken. Follow a healthy and balanced food plan, and be sure your caloric intake doesn't fall too low. You are not going to cause a weight gain or stall by having too few calories.

"I have to eat a lot more calories because I am working out now."

The more you burn, the more you need to eat. This is true, but if you want to lose the junk that's in the trunk, you better stop filling up the caboose with so much juice. I never understood why people flocked to the gyms to work out only to stop off at the juice bar for a smoothie. The kale superfood genie smoothie might have antioxidants and cancer-fighting nutrients that will make you feel healthy. The spinach beet juice extravaganza could put hair on anyone's muscular chest. Your seven-dollar strawberry superfood smoothie has you suckered. People instantly become super stupid and forget when they see certain words like *whole food, natural, organic,* or *superfood*. The 186 calories you burned sitting on the recumbent bike did jack shit.

You see, you are, after all, getting enough calories, and you are not gaining muscle. The bottom line is that with your reduced-calorie allowance for weight loss, you cannot afford an 850-calorie snack. To lose weight, you have to create a caloric deficit—plain and simple. You should not eat back all the calories (or more of the calories) you burned with a high-calorie smoothie snack.

A wise woman once told me that weight loss is 70 percent diet and 30 percent exercise. I can tell you that it is more like 50 percent mind-set, 35 percent diet, and 15 percent exercise. The 15 percent exercise is only because of the metabolic benefits and not the caloric benefits. Do not lose sight of that. Mind-set is everything!

"I can never have the body I used to have before kids. My hips have spread from childbirth."

So often women believe themselves when they say (or think) they can never get their prepregnancy bodies back. They find it much easier to quit or not try. That is the problem. Women have convinced themselves that it is not possible to lose their baby weight. A woman will find her body to be an incomprehensible sight the week after childbirth. New moms going through hormonal changes find this to be less than tolerable.

I agree that covering it up with the biggest sweater and hiding underneath the sweater is much easier than dealing with it. However, if you cover your body up, you will feel worse. Once you have convinced yourself that it is impossible to go back to your prepregnancy state, then you never will. If you decide you will never ever lose the fifty pounds you gained, it is because you decided to eat an excessive amount of calories for nine months.

I laugh at the women who say they cannot get their bodies back because of genetics. Really? I did not know there was a human DNA gene that predisposes a woman never to be able to lose the fifty pounds she gained during her pregnancy.

Here is another good one: "My hips spread from childbirth, and now I have wide hips." Okay, that's a first … Was your baby the size of a full-grown man? I am pretty sure if anyone's hips spread during childbirth, that would mean that her pelvis would shatter, and her baby would not have been able to get out of the ten-centimeter opening.

There is no doubt that having children will jack up your body. There is no doubt it will never be the same. There is no doubt that you will look at yourself in the mirror and cry like a sad soul who will never see her best friend again. There is no doubt that it will be worth every tear. You cannot escape a pregnancy without some damage. I was lucky enough to be blessed with four healthy pregnancies. I gained fifty pounds for each one of my kiddos. *Fifty pounds.* It was not a pretty sight, and I thought my bikini-wearing days were over, but I was not going to allow myself to fall into this trap.

Stop believing that you have to go around wearing loose yoga pants after your baby is born and pack away the maternity clothes. You are done wearing them as soon as your baby is born. Of course, you need to allow your body time to heal and recover from the amazing and very complicated miracle of childbirth, but you shouldn't give it a year … or twenty. Women who blame their long-term weight gain on a pregnancy that occurred several years in the past are no different than a farmer blaming a poor harvest on a drought from ten years prior. Shit or get off the pot already. Donate those maternity dresses before they become your mother-of-the-bride wedding week wardrobe.

I have made my point. Think about the skinny bitch mom in the preschool line. You know, the one with the double stroller and the four-year-old wearing the loose yoga pants. Her hips didn't spread, and neither did yours. Stop believing this bullshit.

"I can't lose weight because of my hormones."

Hormones are the demons of hell. As a mother of four, I can tell you that I was on red-alert-emotional-outcast-watch during all my pregnancies. This lasted until every drop of breast milk was depleted out of my body. I was like a psycho mama bear protecting her young from all evil. One minute I was fine. The next minute I would let my three year old play with razor blades. Then I would freak out and think my ten year old was going to choke on applesauce. If that wasn't bad enough, I had to watch my daughters enter puberty and be affected by these vicious demons.

We have seen it happen: hormones. They can make a normal human crazy. Then when you get older, these hormones affect you even more. At this point, you are used to being a crazy bitch every month. It does not matter that your kids are now hormone-plagued, but now you are going to go through menopause. Menopause is going to happen when it happens. Sure, it is real, but what is not real is all the hog wash about what is going to happen. It will happen if you let it happen. If it does happen, you are in control of it. Don't set yourself up for failure.

I remember being in fifth grade and reading *Dear God, It's Me Margaret* by Judy Blume. I swear I thought my period was coming any day. I had cramps daily. I was bloated. I even thought I was spotting a few times. Exactly three years later I got my period. Yep, approximately 1,095 days of these fake symptoms—the cramps, backaches, headaches, mood swings, and chocolate cravings. Here I am today, counting a total of 156 weeks of listening to all my girlfriends talk about hot flashes and weight gain. More than thirty-six months of lunches filled with complaining about hormones and menopause. A blink of an eye, and my girlfriends have gone from waiting for their first periods to waiting for their last. Anyhow, the shit's all the same. It's going to happen when it's going to happen.

Do not spend the next two thousand days stuffing your face so you can say it's because you are premenopausal. I'm almost fifty, I'm premenopausal, and I refuse to blame my weight gain on hormones. When I gain weight, it is because

I ate too much. That is correct. I was mindlessly stuffing my face with food and acting like the calories didn't count. My jeans became tight because I was sucking down peanut butter by the kilo and pretending my metabolism was broken. My fat ass got fat because I allowed it to happen. I finally stopped gaining weight when I accepted that 50 percent mind-set.

"That's made with a healthy fat, so it's okay to eat it."

This is another true statement, but olive oil still contains one hundred calories per tablespoon. Olive oil is the healthier of the oils. If you soak your vegetables in it, you are still consuming an overabundance of calories in your day.

This is a battle that I have lost many times with my relatives. My family is 100 percent Greek. We come from the land of the olives. My parents were born and raised in Kalamata, Greece. Those Greeks love their oil, which is like liquid gold. The more you use, the healthier you'll be. My mom is an amazing cook, and she loves to cook healthy with home-grown vegetables cooked fresh on the grill. She would serve them and say, "These are healthy. I used a little oil." I thought they tasted delicious, but I would question if I was eating grilled vegetables or some sort of olive oil soup. In terms of calories, the grilled zucchini totaled a full day's worth of calories.

This is true for all healthy fats. Just because a fat is healthy does not mean the calories don't count. I don't care if the butters are grass-fed or the coconut oil, avocado oil, and grapeseed oil are organic. I don't care if the cows are hand-fed with only fed homegrown food. It's still frickin' butter, and it still has calories.

"My friend told me her sister's cousin had a thyroid problem and couldn't lose weight. I think that is my problem."

Blame the ol' thyroid—the goddamn, motherfuckin' thyroid. Seriously, people; let's take a minute to process this. How many times have you thought your thyroid was messed up? How many times have you had it checked? How many times have you been diagnosed with an issue with your thyroid?

Let's play one more game. How many of your friends have a true thyroid issue that has caused weight gain? How many of them lost weight once diagnosed? The lesson here is that even if you do have an issue with your thyroid, it is most likely not the only reason you have junk in the trunk.

Once again, we are back to this simple truth: you eat too much. Put the reality glasses on, and apologize to your thyroid for blaming it for your weight gain. Stop lying to yourself.

"I'm too old to start a program now, and nothing I do will make a difference."

This excuse is one that always baffles me. An older client (who is my age) says that she feels too old to start a program. She feels she can't make improvements due to her age. This is when I have to get real with people. Anyone who thinks they can't make a difference by adding fitness and nutrition into her life at any age is signing up for a shorter life span.

My ninety-eight-year-old grandmother lived longer because of the physical therapy and nutrition that was provided to her. If you are older and retired, going to the gym and participating in a moderate exercise program is better than sitting on the couch all day. Age is just a number. If you think you can't make improvements during your golden years, then you won't. Your body will slow down if you let it;

keep it tuned up, and it will last longer. I have clients who are in their sixties and seventies who could kick anyone's ass, including mine. #JeanNancyandPat #ItsunderhandJon

"I don't have time."

Bullshit. That's all I have to say. I have spent an average of eight hours a day working one-on-one with people over the last twenty years. I have worked with men and women ranging in age from ten to eighty. I have worked with doctors, lawyers, business owners, and superintendents. I have trained artists, firefighters, photographers, musicians, realtors, musicians, teachers, homemakers, and students. My clients all lead busy lives, some busier than others.

Throughout these years, I have listened to the excuses that people have given for various reasons. I concluded that no matter how busy people are, they can always find time to do the things that they make a priority. This caused me to do some self-reflecting. I was busy. I have a husband, four kids, and two dogs. I train more than one hundred clients every week and help thousands each year with nutritional plans. I take life-coaching classes, I have an online business, I train the local fire department, and I run ultramarathons.

I still managed to find time write this book because it was something that was important to me.

My clients who claim they don't have time to cook always show up to their sessions with perfectly manicured nails. It is those same people who manage to watch every series on Netflix known to man because that was important to them. I am not knocking those things, as I think it is important to do things that you enjoy. I am merely pointing out the fact that making this way of life important can easily become a priority.

Once you bump health and wellness to the top, then everything else will fall into place. No matter how busy people are, they can always find time to do the things they make a priority.

That's it! Three simple rules. If you follow these Golden Girlfriend Survival Rules, you will make it to the nearest safety station. These safety stations are the sanity areas that we will visit throughout this wellness journey. Safety stations are like aid stations in the middle of a dark forest that you need to get to in order to survive. At the safety stations, you can catch your breath, regroup, and talk sense into yourself. But you first have to follow the survival rules to get to the safety stations, so you can receive the survival equipment that you need to continue.

5

What's the Point?
Keeping It Real

I n order for this to work, you need to be real. You need to be accountable to yourself. Often when we view things on an abstract level, we distort the view. This means you need to put things in a concrete realm and see things in black-and-white; otherwise, you will fall into a state of denial. This is a professional way of saying, "You are kidding yourself, so get your head out of your ass before you weigh a million pounds and need medical attention."

I know that is harsh, but it does hold some truth. You would not believe the fucked-up head games people play with themselves when it comes to the scale. It is the most jacked up thing ever. For as many smart people I know, I have seen the IQ of an individual plummet twenty or thirty points when it comes to bathroom scale logic. It's actually quite humorous.

Bathroom Scale Logic

I have memories of scale manipulation when I first began trying to lose weight. In high school, I had gained weight by eating too many Suzy Qs. It was in the eighties. I remember it like it was yesterday with Aqua Net plastered all over the floral wallpaper, and hot-pink lipstick stains on the goldenrod bathroom sink. My parents had one of those scales that had a dial. I always made sure that the little line was just to the left of the zero when I got on so I could be just a little under my actual weight. I always had some legitimate justification for this. My hair was wet, or I was wearing earrings. Whatever it was, I needed to give myself those extra little dashes on the scale every single day. The ironic thing was that if my hair was actually ever wet or if I was having my period, there was no way I would even think about walking past the scale, let alone get on it.

Then there were the times I would get on it and not like what I saw. God forbid the scale was up a pound because I stuffed my face with another Suzy Q the day before. I would move the scale around the bathroom until I saw the number I wanted to see. Oh yes, I did. Often this would take fifteen or more minutes. I would tilt it, flip it, or move it to the kitchen. I would move it to the bedroom, put it on the carpet, and even play with the way it sat on the bathroom tiles. Each time I got a different weight, but I would keep going until I got the number I wanted. Once I did, I could move on with my day as if none of this even happened. I had forgotten all about the original weigh-in, as well as the Suzy Q I ate the night before.

Then there were the mornings when moving the scale wasn't enough. I had to go into level II advanced scale manipulation techniques. This is when you get on the scale using different mounting strategies: tiptoes, flat-footed, feet wide, toes closed, one foot first, then the other. Getting on the scale and then jumping off quickly while supporting my weight on the bathroom sink. These are all examples of scale denial.

For a while, I would even weigh myself with clothes and shoes on because then I would never know what I really weighed. I did this for several weeks in a row. It dawned on me that I had an average weight of what I was with shoes and clothes on, and that became my expectation. I thought back to moving the scale around in my parents' bathroom and getting on the scale with tippy-toes. I did this to create a number that was inaccurate enough to please me for the day.

Weight is just a number. This was a life-changing epiphany for me. I mean, we know this ... We do ... but we still let the number somehow consume us. No matter how hard we try and no matter what we say, we let that damn number dictate our lives.

There are many new habits I want you to create. One of them is learning that the number on the scale should not control you. Having the number on the scale determine how you perceive yourself means that you are walking a very fine line between practicing mental wellness and developing an unhealthy obsession with the scale, which can cause more harm than good. This will only lead to a distorted reality of your true progress.

With all joking aside, eating disorders are nothing to play around with. These habits are ones that could lead to others that could become dangerous or unhealthy. These kinds of obsessive-compulsive habits could lead to other dangerous or unhealthy habits. If you feel that moving the scale around sixteen times until you see the number you want isn't doing you any harm, you could be wrong.

This is going to change right now. Hold on. I am going to restate that: *this is going to change right now.* You are a role model not only for your children but for everyone watching you rock this program. Start right now by understanding that the scale is a guide and that you will see the numbers fluctuate. My point is that you will see the results you want with persistence and consistency.

I would like to share a story of a woman who I worked with and who suffered from severe scale denial. She ended up in a self-sabotaging disaster resulting in a damaged metabolism.

Lynn always struggled with weighing herself. She would often let the number on the scale lead the direction of her entire day. She would wake up feeling great about herself and the food choices that she made the day before. If she weighed herself and the scale showed even the slightest weight gain, she would lose her shit. She would become angry, sad, irrational, and sometimes even go psycho. It was not good. Lynn knew she had to get better at this or it would be her demise. She had to learn to accept the daily fluctuations that occur in the human body. After working on this difficult mental task, she got much better at it. Yet, she learned to manipulate the system.

The best time to weigh yourself is the very first thing in the morning after you have gone to the bathroom. This would usually work fine, except on mornings when Lynn couldn't go. On those poopless mornings, Lynn wouldn't weigh herself. We all know that eating a Babe Ruth bar the night before could cause at least a one-pound weight gain, but Lynn couldn't handle seeing that extra weight.

Then there would be days when Lynn wouldn't eat or drink anything until she pooped. Once duty called, she would rush to the bathroom, strip down to nothing, and get on the scale. Interestingly, the later in the day she weighed herself, the lower the number would be. This was the best discovery ever. Lynn struck gold when she found this out. She started weighing herself later in the morning every day. These numbers would make the birds chirp and the rainbows appear over her house.

Lynn figured out that when she sweat, the number on the scale would go down even more. She threw that in the mix as well. She included a workout without drinking any water, as the water would add to the scale.

The more she sweat, the less she weighed. It was the best. This (fake) weight loss would ensure the presence of birds and rainbows every day. Life was good—so she thought.

In reality, Lynn was putting her body in an extreme state of dehydration so she could see this invalid number on the scale. In reality, she was not losing weight. She was losing water. The scale was showing a number that was about five pounds less than her actual weight. Lynn was going several hours without nutrition or hydration every single day just to catch a mere glimpse of this fantasy number. This behavior did not show what Lynn weighed, and it didn't show whether Lynn was making progress on the program. Lynn continued to engage in this behavior around the scale for months and months, which ended up doing serious irreversible damage to her kidneys and metabolism.

Lynn even justified this behavior by telling herself that she had enough calories left in her day so she could afford it. Lynn couldn't have been more wrong. When Lynn had to go for a doctor's appointment, she would go that extra mile and avoid food or water until after the weigh-in with the nurse. It didn't matter if the appointment was at four o'clock in the afternoon. Maybe she would eat something that didn't weigh much, but she needed to get on that scale and see the lowest possible number. The problem was that after her weigh-ins, whether at the doctor or at home, she would be so hungry that she would inevitably overeat

Essentially, Lynn was teaching her metabolism to slow down by skipping meals—no food for dinner until after she worked out and pooped the next day. Cheese crackers, pudding, nuggets, fries, PBJ, BLT, OMG, WTF! Lynn had destroyed her metabolism, which ended up taking years to repair. Now that her metabolism was moving as slow as a fucking one-hundred-year-old bullfrog, she had eaten enough food to feed an orphanage. Lynn had to work that much harder to repair the damage she had done to her body with her behavior on her bathroom scale. #nomorebullfrog

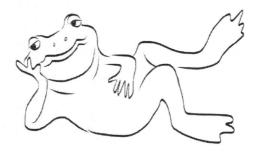

You see, the point here is health and wellness. The big picture is that the scale will move if you do all the right things. Starving yourself, not drinking water, and moving the scale around are all poor habits. Standing on your head while weighing yourself will not reduce the amount of fat that you have on your body, and it will not lower your body weight or stabilize your blood sugars. These obsessive behaviors will not give you good heart health, build muscle, or nourish your body, and they won't provide the vitamins and minerals needed to make you stronger. That is the point.

The point is not to ever let the scale have power over you. It is a guide. It is simply a way to measure yourself; it has no way of knowing how much water you drank or how much sodium was in your meal from the night before. The number you see is simply an approximate reference to how you are progressing. If you have been following your program and doing everything according to plan and the scale moves up, then you know it is merely a fluctuation. When this happens, it is very important that you go through the following steps to secure your power over the scale:

Bathroom Scale Inner Strength Test

1. Ask yourself the following questions: "Have I done anything to cause this weight fluctuation to occur?" and/or "Have I exhibited any behaviors that would cause a weight gain at this time?" If you answered no, then move on to the next step.

2. You are probably in the bathroom, so look in the mirror and say the following out loud (it has to be out loud or it won't work): "If I am doing everything

right and the scale is not moving or moving in the wrong direction, it will eventually move, and I have nothing to worry about. It is the big picture that matters. I will not let the scale control me."

3. Then I want you to think about all the progress you have made and how unrealistic it is to think that you actually gained fat for no reason. When you feel your heart smiling again, move on the step 4.

4. Look at the scale, and give it a hand gesture of your choice. This will vary depending on your state of mind, age group, and level of frustration. No one will see you do this, so have fun with it.

5. Look in the mirror one last time, and tell yourself that you are going to have a fabulous day!

Over the years, many of my clients initially laugh when I ask them to perform this bathroom scale inner strength test, but the ones who do eventually change their mind-set into one that is more realistic. *It is the big picture that matters.* This is not a contest, and there is no rush to the finish line. The goal is to get healthy safely, without issues, and to cross the line without ever worrying about needing to start over.

Be Accurate on Your Calculations

When we do mindless things, we don't make ourselves accountable for our actions. We only take credit for all of our hard work, and we forget about the splurges we take. Everybody does this from time to time, and until you start paying attention to your behaviors, you will continue to fool yourself. At the end of the day, you need to count every strawberry and grape you ate because they count. You have to take accountability for your actions. You can't burn calories *thinking* about going for that walk when you *almost* went on it. You also need to count the calories you sucked down when you polished off your son's triple-thick milkshake. You may justify the five sips as *well deserved*, but at 1,100 calories a shake, that will add up to quite a bit.

These miscalculations have led to our demise. It is the bullfrog within all of us that drags us down—the negative, pessimistic, downer-like behaviors that we have all misconceived as broken metabolisms. A bullfrog doesn't recall all the hours she spends lying around on her lily pad doing nothing all day. She only counts the hard work that she has to do to catch a few flies for dinner. In her mind, she amplifies her hard work and perceives that she has worked harder than she actually has. A bullfrog also forgets to count all the flies and insects that she mindlessly gobbles down all day long while her ugly tadpoles are at frog school. She ends her day thinking she has barely eaten and endlessly complains at the bus stop about how she just can't lose weight.

The saddest part about this story is that this bullfrog is super ugly, and she has no idea how mindless her behaviors are. Unless she takes time to self-reflect and educate herself, she will never succeed in weight loss. I would have loved to helped this bullfrog, but she needs to help herself before anyone can help her. That, and she doesn't like me. #idontlikeher #noonelikesher

Look at the Big Picture

If you were building your dream home, you would envision the finished product. You would fantasize about hosting dinner parties in your beautiful kitchen and opening Christmas presents in front of your beautiful fireplace. You would see the Pinterest image of your home and look forward to moving in, knowing all the hard work that still lies ahead.

When you plan your wedding, get a college degree, or save for a vacation you do the same. Why is it that we don't do this when we take on the enormous project of reconstructing our lifestyles?

When building a home, do you quit halfway through because you are frustrated that something didn't run as planned during the drywall phase? Do you abandon the project completely because of a rainy summer and a delay in the concrete work? Why do we do this time and time again when we diet? It is the same thing, people. You are spending all of this time, money, and energy on a huge project and then abandoning ship because something goes wrong. You leave it. You don't look back. The house sits there abandoned until you decide to build a new one, and then you have to start over ... again. Do you see how stupid and ridiculous this is?

Let's go back to building your dream home. If something goes wrong, you realistically would take the time to figure it out. Do not let the scale derail you. Use it as a guide, but do not let it control you. It may delay things a bit, but you would eventually have your finished product. Does it matter if you move in this year or next year? In the end, you will have your house, and it will be the way you want it. If you keep abandoning it, you will never see the finished product. If it takes you ten times longer to move into this new home, then so be it. You will be happy, and it will be worth the wait.

With weight loss, you have to go into a program with the mind-set that there is no timeline. This cannot be predicted, and it cannot be expected. You must look at the big picture and visualize the end result—not just the Pinterest physical result but the internal and emotional result that you will feel. It's the gift of health and wellness that you will live with endlessly.

6

Your New Plan: Starting the Day Right

There are so many different health-and-wellness philosophies and programs. Let's say you won an all-inclusive two-week vacation anywhere in the world, and you could to pick where you wanted to go. It would be hard to pick. You could make a quick choice with a little research based on other people's experiences. Now, instead, let's suppose you are told you have to make this decision quickly and that you have to live there forever. That changes things, right? Now that you are supposed to pick a vacation destination as a permanent place of residence, you will be a lot more cautious about your decision and take your time deciding where you would want to go.

The same is true about choosing your eating plan. Do not look at your eating plan as a temporary program. This is the problem! The marketing giants of the dieting world draw you in by telling their bull-crap stories, how easy their plan is, and how you will not have to change your lifestyle. We have all been sucked into this, and I have been guilty of it too—not just for weight loss. Any informercial can talk anyone into buying anything with three easy payments. There is no such thing as easy—*initially*.

Initially, practicing a new lifestyle will be difficult, but then it becomes easy. Once your new health behaviors become second nature, like a habit, you will become good at implementing the new behaviors. This should be your goal. This is true for many things in life.

The first time your hairstylist held a pair of scissors in her hands in beauty school, she didn't have grace and confidence, but now she styles your hair like a pro as she chops away without even looking. She cuts as she yaps about her dumb brother-in-law and stupid neighbor who she can't stand. Same goes for you on the first day that you brought your baby home from the hospital. You were nervous as shit that you may do something wrong. I'm sure you're a bit more confident now. You are going to have to accept the fact that you are going back to kindergarten.

Starting with the basics is the best way to ease into a realistic program. I promise if you stick with this new program as outlined word for word in this book, you will think that following your new meal plan will eventually be pretty easy. So, find a plan you can learn to love and stay with for years to come.

One thing I find very frustrating is that over the years, there have been so many different types of diets. How did this come about? The human body is a very complex and detailed machine. As complicated as it is, there is only one way to lose weight, even though there are many ways to trick your body into losing weight. Sustaining that loss while living your life without gaining it all back is the hard part. Unless a realistic plan is chosen, individuals have a 5 percent chance of keeping their weight off once it is lost. You are one of the ninety-five people out of one hundred who have gained back the weight you lost on one of those weight-loss plans, but not this time because this is the *last first day* on a diet.

So why all the different diets? Weight Watchers, Atkins, South Beach, and keto. Paleo, Dukan, The Zone, HCG, Whole 30, low carb, vegan, high protein, ultralow fat, and intermittent fasting. Why this outrageous desire to have a name for their diet? What the fuck is that about? You didn't get a goddamn dog, so you don't need to name it.

Let's start with that. You are going to eat right—the way you should—and you are not going to set yourself up for failure by joining a frickin' cult and being part of a community of diet followers like these people who have to go around preaching the praises of Dr. Atkins or wearing tank tops that say "Vegans do it better." I'm sorry … You do not need to join a fraternity to lose weight.

Don't get me wrong. I understand the sense of community thing. The bottom line is that you are doing this to better your health. You should not have to pick a diet so you can fit into a group. For example, you may like the guidelines of the paleo diet, but the diet does not allow peanuts, a legume. Most people don't even know what a fucking legume is. The paleo wannabes stop sucking down peanut butter for a few weeks, so they can post about it on the paleo blog and feel like they fit in. Meanwhile, they have no idea why they are eliminating peanuts from their diet and end up always blowing the entire program because they really don't understand it.

What if you like eating a plant-based but also enjoy chicken? Then do it! It doesn't have to have a name. I call this *nutritional plan confusion*. It's when you don't know how you want others to identify you in the world of nutrition. You feel like you have to have a name for your food plan. Guess what … You don't! You are eating clean and healthy. As you start losing weight, people will ask you how you did it. It is still very awkward for me, as I have to tell them that I eat the way humans are intended to eat. I usually get a blank look followed by a list of questions such as: "So, low carb? Keto? Atkins?" It astonishes me to this day. It proves that people have a direct correlation between losing weight and a marketed program.

Marketed … or free.

Target.

On your head.

Get it?

This time, you are not selecting a program. You are going to learn how to eat the way our bodies are intended to eat. We have to reprogram your system and reboot everything. Somehow over the years, we have been corrupted by society and the things in our world that make our lives convenient and easy. We have been brainwashed to think that it is easier to order out and buy a prepackaged meal than it is to make one at home. We have become lazy, and this has cost us our health.

Your new food program will not only include a healthier diet, but it will also create a healthier world for you and your family. If you are feeling a bit uneasy about the fact that your new diet doesn't have a name, you should. It's the only one of its kind. It's the kind that you're not on. It's just called *the way you eat*.

You should construct each meal with certain amounts of nutrients to create a balanced meal. The amounts and portions will depend on each individual. That part is up to you to figure out. I will be referring to these categories as *the three must-haves*. You need to have all three of these macronutrients in every meal. Learn to incorporate these foods and the approximate amounts into every single one of your meals, including snacks.

Before your head explodes, I need to remind you that you are still in kindergarten. We are going to start learning this slow. Don't go getting all psycho OCD on me yet with your macronutrient calculator and food scale. Remember that it was just yesterday that you were scoffing down apple cider donuts like they were never being sold in North America ever again.

Must-Haves

Protein

20–25 grams will help sustain your hunger until you can eat again. Start your day with a meal that will stimulate your brain cells. Your metabolism will start moving and keep you satisfied longer.

+ eggs or egg whites
+ protein shake or smoothie
+ protein bar
+ Greek yogurt
+ tofu
+ any meat or fish

+ milk or alternative milk, such as soy, almond, or coconut milk

+ cottage cheese

Complex Carbohydrates

With 30–40 grams of complex carbs, you will give your blood sugar and insulin levels a spike. This will give you a bit of energy. This is not to be confused with 5-Hour Energy, which is a stimulant. A carbohydrate will give your muscles a boost and give you a kick in your step. Many foods have hundreds of grams of carbohydrates. Your body will mostly likely not burn that many carbs but will turn them to fat, which I will explain later. For now, try to keep your breakfast carbs at about 30–40 grams. This is not very much, but it is plenty.

+ oats

+ grits

+ farina

+ quinoa

+ cereal

+ toast

+ pancake or waffle (without syrup)

+ healthy muffin

Healthy Fat

You should eat about 8–10 grams of a healthy fat in each meal. As much as I love bacon, I would be a liar if I told you it is a healthy fat. Healthy fats are called monosaturated fats— you know, the ones that don't cause heart disease and stroke. Blah, blah, blah … the boring ones. No cheese, no butter, no lard, and no fucking bacon either. I am not saying you can't have a lard and bacon sandwich ever again, but I am saying that it's not considered healthy. Ain't my rule, but I can tell you that there are many amazing and wonderful fats that are healthy. Thank the Lord on this one. Every breakfast should include one serving of a healthy fat as well.

+ avocado

+ avocado oil

+ olives

+ olive oil

+ grape seed oil

+ egg yolk

+ coconut

+ coconut oil

+ nuts

+ nut butter

Now looking at the foods listed, I am certain you can mix and match them to create quite a few breakfast options. Keep in mind that you do not need to have all three categories represented in each breakfast. An ideal breakfast will have adequate levels of protein, carbohydrates, and fats. If you are counting grams and freaking out right now, *relax* … You are in kindergarten. All you need to do is select one item from each category and move on.

If you are calculating carbohydrates versus protein, then you need to walk up to the chalkboard and put your name on the detention list. Not allowed. Let's start by creating some things to eat for breakfast without getting college-level scientific with your Cheerios.

Here are some of my favorite breakfast choices. If you notice, there are some extras that do not fall into a category. Take a breath and eat the meal. Later on, I will identify where fruit and other items fall. For now, eat your damn breakfast before you miss the fucking kindergarten bus.

Breakfast

Start your day with breakfast every morning. So often, people say they can't do breakfast, or they don't have time for it. Breakfast is one of the most important meals of the day. It sets you up for success for the entire morning. You are breaking the fast by giving your body food and having a few hundred calories to get your system started after hours of fasting through the night. Believe it or not, when your body is asleep, your metabolism slows down, as it is not stimulated with food. Once awake, you are burning calories. If you don't give your body any nutrients, your metabolism will remain in its slow-moving state.

When you break the fast and provide nutrition to your moving body, your metabolism will start moving. It starts burning more calories throughout the day, giving you a better functioning metabolic rate.

Don't be confused with the type of breakfast that you should have. We are not Laura Ingalls Wilder. We do not live in *Little House on the Prairie*. Back then, Ma made a full, hearty breakfast with eggs and bacon. There was potato hash, grits, biscuits, and gravy every morning. You do not have to go to such an extent to have breakfast. All you need to do is break your fast by eating a few hundred calories to get your system started. You have a multitude of options to pick from, and you won't even have to spend a lot of time preparing them.

Right away, people have to go to their gun belts and pull out their rifles loaded with excuses for why they can't have breakfast. So often people say they can't do breakfast or they don't have time for it. I spent decades thinking I didn't need it either. I can bet that at one point in your life you were also guilty of being a nonbreakfast eater.

Despite all the bullshit excuses you gave yourself and everyone else, the bottom line was that you figured you would save yourself the calories. Why eat while you're half sleeping and rushing out the door? You want to save those calories so you can mindlessly shove food down your throat at night when no one is watching.

How do I know you do this? You see, I skipped breakfast for years. My thinking was exactly like that of Shawna's. I am sharing her story, as many of you may find it helpful.

> Shawna never had to worry about her weight before. Now that she was working again and no longer stayed home with her kids, she noticed that her clothes were a bit tight and her weight had crept up a bit. Not knowing what to do to get it under control, she decided to start logging her food and

keeping track of her calories. According to the app she downloaded, she was told that she should eat 1,550 calories each day. That seemed like plenty. As Shawna began entering everything she ate into her log, she found that she often ate more than her 1,550-calorie limit by several hundred calories each day. She did some research and learned how to omit certain foods to get her calorie levels closer to her goal. In the end, she enjoyed her wine at dinner, and her sweet tooth splurges were something she couldn't live without.

One morning she overslept and didn't have a chance to make her morning oats with berries and almond butter. As stressed as she was, she was able to drink a few cups of coffee with sugar-free sweetener to get her through the morning. That day when she logged her lunch, she noticed she had about 400 extra calories to spare for the day because she skipped her breakfast meal.

The light bulb went on, and the skipping of breakfast began.

Shawna didn't have the extra minute and forty-five seconds that it took to put the oatmeal in the microwave and walk away while she brushed her teeth. She no longer had time in the morning to mix in the almond butter and berries as she made her kids their cereal. She also did not have the three minutes that she used to have to eat the oatmeal. She still scrolled through Facebook wasting time until the bus came to pick up her kids, so she could take a shower and leave for work. Instead of having a healthy breakfast, Shawna convinced herself that she didn't have time for this important meal that would enhance her metabolism and keep her from overeating.

You see, Shawna found a loophole. She found a way to say breakfast did not work for her, so she could skip it and eat those calories later in the day. This is one of many excuses people give for not eating breakfast. People will say they aren't hungry. They claim nothing looks good. They say they read that skipping breakfast will help you lose weight. Wrong … Those same people will mindlessly eat little handfuls of miscellaneous things throughout the day. They don't consider that eating (Girlfriend Survival Rule 3, Lie 1).

Shawna, much like many other people, told herself how she didn't eat much. She told her friends that she was not eating enough calories (Girlfriend Survival Rule 3, Lie 3). Shawna swore she did not get hungry and never ate. This is because Shawna did not actually put food on a plate throughout the day and have a meal. Yet, the 1,387 calories she had consumed throughout the day added up. This caused Shawna not to feel hungry until much later in the day. At that point, Shawna had set herself up with the misconception that she had not eaten. She then thought she could eat what she wanted. From the second she walked in the door until she went to bed, her mouth was in constant chewing motion. At this point, poor planning and hunger resulted in full permission to lose control. This is when mishmash eating occurs.

To make you feel better, I am going to give you an example of one of my mishmash predinner food fiascos. To start, I would eat a few handfuls of every ingredient that was in my dinner recipe. At the same time, I would have almonds because I heard those were good to tide me over before a meal. Bites of cheese, nibbles of bread, even spoonfuls of tomato sauce. As I cooked, I made the kids' lunches for the next day. I'd eat a few chips, some peanut butter, a few corners of sandwiches, and even a broken cookie.

Then it was dinnertime. I would eat my meal and whatever the kids didn't eat. I would say to myself, "What's with the kids anyway? Who in their right mind doesn't finish a perfectly good bowl of macaroni and cheese? One or two bites … That's nothing." This would go on throughout the cleanup and into the night. Every night … me, you, and Shawna.

So here I had mindlessly consumed thousands of calories that I had completely forgotten about. Later I would blame unexplained weight gain on unrealistic mythical factors. Should I blame my hormones or my faulty thyroid? You see, there is nothing wrong with your metabolism. The problem is your mind-set. You are starving, and you need to start with breakfast. I am going to help you come up with some realistic breakfast choices so you can start to incorporate these choices as your first meal of the day.

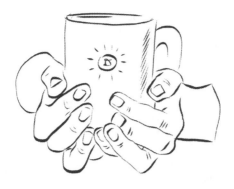

Breakfast Ideas

Bangin' Blueberry Blitz

    1 cup Greek yogurt

    1/2 cup blueberries

    2 teaspoons ground flaxseed

    5 walnut halves, chopped

    agave

Spoon yogurt in a small bowl and add toppings. Drizzle with agave as desired.

Green Getufit Shake

    1 serving protein powder

    1 cup almond milk

1 tablespoon peanut butter (or nut butter)

1/2 avocado

1 tablespoon flaxseeds

handful spinach

ice

Add all ingredients to blender and blend until smooth. Pour into your favorite tall glass.

Getufit Avocado Toast

English muffin, sliced

1/2 avocado

1 slice of tomato

1 egg cooked the way you want

Toast English muffin and top with avocado, tomato, and egg.

Cereal Celebration

1 cup Fiber One or Kashi cereal

1 cup milk of choice

1/2 cup blueberries

20 almonds

Getufit Omelet

> 4 egg whites and 1 full egg
>
> handful of spinach or veggie of choice
>
> side of avocado

Quinoa Avocado Egg Bowl

> 1/2 cup cooked quinoa
>
> 1/2 avocado sliced
>
> 1 egg cooked the way you want
>
> hot sauce or feta (optional)

Chocolate Dream Smoothie

> 1 serving chocolate protein powder
>
> 1 cup almond milk
>
> 2 tablespoon PB2
>
> 1 tablespoon unsweetened cocoa
>
> ice

Add all ingredients to blender and blend until smooth.
Pour into your favorite tall glass.

Quinoa Blueberry Bowl

1/2 cup raw quinoa

1 cup unsweetened vanilla almond milk

1/2 cup fresh or frozen blueberries

cinnamon (optional)

Cook quinoa on stovetop by bringing milk to boil and adding quinoa. Simmer until cooked, about 20 minutes. Top with blueberries and cinnamon.

BLT

1 egg cooked the way you want

1 wedge Laughing Cow cheese

1 slice turkey bacon

sliced tomato

lettuce

1 corn or flour tortilla or 2 slices toast

Layer ingredients and wrap up in the tortilla or sandwich between slices of toast.

Now that you have all this amazing information, you have to put it to good use. Reading about it and saying you're going to do it will not count. If you don't want to sit down and eat an actual meal, do what I do … Eat your breakfast on the go, which you can do in many different ways. You can eat it as you get ready for work. You can graze on it as you sit there and yell at your kids to get their asses out the door so they don't miss the bus. You can also chomp on it while you watch the moms at the bus stop gossiping about everyone who isn't there, including you. You could actually take a whole flippin' three minutes and eat it like a normal person.

Newsflash: You're Not That Busy

You would like to think you are. You can tell yourself, and anyone else who pretends to give a shit, that you are so goddamn busy that you can't sit down to eat your motherfucking breakfast. Instead, you stand at the window spooning cereal into your mouth all while you are trying to read the lips of Mackenzie Dunlap's mom as she stands there looking all put together in her pantsuit. She's ready to conquer the world at her nine-to-five job, and you wonder if she eats breakfast. If she can do it, you can too.

Today is the last day that you will cheat yourself out of this meal. If you choose to pretend you don't have time to eat it, then make sure you fit it in somewhere in your morning. Drink a shake in the car. Eat a bar on the train. Meet Mackenzie's mom for a damn bowl of oatmeal. She can tell you how she fits it all in since you're on chapter 6 of this book and you are still sitting there wondering how you're going to do this. Fucking Mackenzie's mom …

7

Lunchtime: Feeding Time at the Zoo ...

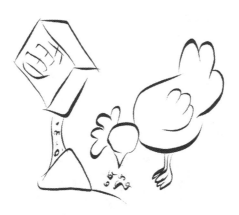

Lunch is everyone's favorite. Usually, lunchtime comes with a break. Usually. Somehow lunch is labeled as the break that everyone has to take to refuel with food. It's the middle of the day meal. The midday brain break. The halfway point in your day when you finally get to eat something and regroup for the rest of the day. Even Fred Flintstone waited for the bell to ring at the Slate Rock and Gravel Company. He would dart off to suck down his brontosaurus burger, and then he would head back to the rock quarry for more labor-intensive work. Even in the Stone Age people got a lunchtimes. It's what we do … no matter how long ago and no matter where we live. This important meal should not be taken for granted or abused. It's not one that is often skipped, but it is one that is abused.

It is like feeding time at the frickin' zoo. Watch out, motherfuckers, because at the strike of twelve o'clock, the drive-through lanes will be at full capacity. Those poor fast-food employees must hate this time of day with a passion. Hungry people in a massive hurry to get their food the way they want it in less than sixty seconds. Don't forget all the fixings on the side and a large Diet Coke. Meanwhile, the CEOs of these companies are dining on yachts someplace in the south of France. Their brilliant dollar menu idea was a gold mine. Pharmaceutical reps are retiring young due to sales of medications.

Feeding time at the zoo ...

How the heck does one abuse lunch?

"Hamburgers, Filet-O-Fish, cheeseburgers, french fries, icy drinks, thick shakes, sundaes, apple pies."

This is how.

Have you even been to any restaurant between the hours of 11:00 a.m. and 2:00 p.m.? The drive-through line is dozens of cars deep. The lobbies of sit-down franchises are flipping tables and burgers faster than most people can spell the words: *lazy fat ass who can't just pack a lunch.*

Sorry, but that's what it boils down to. People then come to me bitching and complaining that they have no time to make lunch. They have no time to shop for food items to bring a lunch to work. They have no time think about the planning that it takes to make a list. They have no time to go to the store, make a goddamn sandwich, throw it in a fucking bag, and bring it to work.

Really?

I would challenge any of these people to set a timer every single Monday through Friday. Start timing. See how much time it takes you and your dumb coworkers to decide where you are going to go eat, who is going to drive, and which route you are going to take. How long until you get there, park your car in the overflowing parking lot, walk across the lot, and then wait in a line longer than the Mississippi. It's true ... but for lunch, you and everyone else will wait.

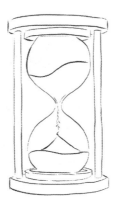

Your imaginary timer is still ticking.

You wait for them to get your food wrong.

Your coworker's order is completely missing.

The bill has been jacked up.

Six minutes remain to actually eat.

You decide not to count the calories from the cheese on your salad because you didn't actually order it.

Since you didn't eat all the lettuce, it will offset the calories from the fries you ate from your friend's tray.

But wait.

The timer still ticks as you race back to work.

While not getting much of a break because you have convinced yourself you don't have time to make a lunch.

The saddest part of this scenario is that you have done this. I have done this. Millions of people do it every single day … which is fine in a world where it doesn't affect our health and wellness. In a world full of calories and large portions, it is contributing to the fact that *we have become lazy asses* and need to start packing lunches. Don't get me wrong; going out for an occasional lunch can be fun and enjoyable. To make this new world of yours one that you can live in forever, eating a homemade lunch is one that should be part of your routine.

By the way, the average person wastes more than four hours each week getting to and from a lunch destination during the day. They spend an average of $42.78 a week on food. They consume an average of 834 calories a day on lunch. That equals 16,680 calories a month for lunches during the week. I'm pretty sure the 16 hours spent each month and $171.12 can make a lot of fabulous lunches. This would save you time, money, and calories.

Here are some healthy lunch options that you could throw together for lunch. Refer to the *must-haves* noted earlier to be sure you include a protein, carbohydrate, and fat in each meal. As a reminder, portions and caloric amounts will differ from person to person. These meals can be created with different portion sizes to accommodate individual needs.

Lunch Ideas

Turkey Apple Cheddar Melt

2 slices whole-wheat bread

2 teaspoons whole-grain mustard, divided

1/2 medium apple, sliced

2 ounces low-sodium deli turkey*

2 tablespoons shredded cheddar cheese, divided

1 cup mixed greens

Top one slice of bread with 1 teaspoon mustard, apple, turkey, and 1 tablespoon cheese. Top the other slice of bread with the remaining 1 teaspoon mustard and 1 tablespoon cheese. Toast sandwich halves faceup in a toaster oven until the cheese begins to melt and bubble. Add the mixed greens to the sandwich before serving.

*Look for a deli turkey with less than 150 milligrams sodium per 1-ounce serving.

Turkey and Pear Pita

1/2 large whole-wheat pita round (save the other half for another meal)

3 1/2 ounces low-sodium deli turkey

1/2 medium pear, sliced

2 tablespoons shredded cheddar cheese

1 cup mixed greens

Include all ingredients into the pita and enjoy.

Chicken Pita

1/2 cup chopped romaine

1/2 cup sliced cucumber

1/4 cup grated carrot

4 ounces chicken

1/2 large whole-wheat pita round, toasted

1/4 cup hummus

Combine greens, cucumber, carrot, chicken, and hummus. Add to pita and enjoy.

Awesome Apple Chicken Salad

mixed greens

4 ounces chicken

1/2 cup chopped apple

1/2 cup strawberries

1/4 cup slivered almonds

2 tablespoons light dressing

Layer greens, chicken, apple, and strawberries in a bowl and top with almonds and dressing.

Holy Hummus

1/2 cup chopped romaine

1/2 cup sliced cucumber

1/4 cup grated carrot

1/2 large whole-wheat pita round, toasted

2 tablespoons hummus

1/4 cup beans of choice

Combine greens, cucumber, and carrot. Mix beans and hummus. Add to pita and enjoy.

Perfect Salmon Avocado Pita

2 slices avocado

2 slices tomato

2–4 ounces smoked or canned salmon (or chicken)

1 tablespoon light mayo

2 corn tortillas

Lightly brown 2 corn tortillas (optional but yummy), add half of ingredients to each tortilla, and fold into 2 pitas.

Oriental Chicken Salad

mixed greens

3–6 ounces grilled chicken or fish

1/2 cup canned mandarin oranges

2 tablespoons pecans

2 tablespoons light ginger dressing

2 tablespoons shelled edamame

Layer chicken, oranges, and pecans on top of romaine and top with pecans and dressing.

All-American BLT

2–4 ounces chicken (grilled or canned)

2 toasted corn tortillas or choice of bread (200-calorie maximum)

1 tablespoon light olive oil mayo (optional)

1 slice turkey bacon

sliced tomato

lettuce

mustard (optional)

other veggies (optional)

Combine ingredients. Add to bread/pita or tortilla and enjoy. Serve with small garden salad, carrots, or light yogurt.

Greek Cottage Cheese Surprise

(Try this … even if you don't think you will like!)

1 cup cottage cheese (any fat percentage)

1/2 cup chopped cucumber

1/2 cup chopped tomato

chopped onion (optional)

olives (optional)

2 ounces chopped chicken breast

2 tablespoons light balsamic vinaigrette

oregano

Combine cottage cheese, veggies, chicken, and dressing and mix well. Top with oregano. Opahhhhh.

Bangin' Beet Salad

mixed greens

3–6 ounces grilled chicken or fish

1/2 cup chopped pickled beets

2 tablespoons pecans

2 tablespoons light dressing

2 tablespoons goat cheese or feta

Prepare bed of mixed greens and top with remaining ingredients.

Is your stomach sending messages to your brain telling it to get your shit together? Are you wanting to make some of these fabulous lunches? I'm guessing that it is. I am also willing to bet that after you're done reading for the day, you have some reason for why you don't have time to shop or prepare these lunches. Since we both know that is going to happen, I am going to save you the humiliation of having to explain to yourself (or anyone else you have blabbed to).

Before you convince yourself that you will start this diet next week, let's ease into this. You have to eat lunch tomorrow. It doesn't have to be my Fancy, Dancy Beet Salad or the Sha-Sha Chicken Apple Blah-Blah Wrap. It also doesn't have to be the triple-cheese crap-burger and chicken fries you normally get. It doesn't matter what you eat tomorrow, but it should have all three of the must-haves. It should ideally come from home. I realize that you will need to eat out from time to time. We will learn how to make wise choices in these situations. In the beginning, understanding everything you are putting in your mouth will establish habits that will help you in the long run.

8

A Long Time Until Dinner: Combating the Gargoyles

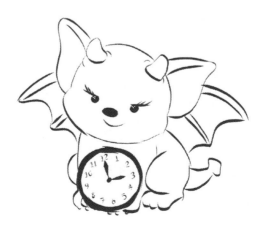

It seems like breakfasts and lunches are the safest of the meals. Something happens after three or four o'clock in the afternoon. No matter who you are or where you live, no matter your age or your gender, when the clock strikes three o'clock, your brain gets taken over by these invisible monsters. They take over your ability to make logical food decisions. Don't laugh. These little fuckers are perched on your shoulder. They just sit, waiting for this witching hour to surface. They are little gargoyles lined up, planning the way they are going to fog your brain. They watch you eat an ungodly amount of shit for the next three or four hours. They watch you eat until you hate yourself more than you did the night before when you swore you wouldn't do it again.

Witching Hour

noun

1. the time late at night when the powers of a witch, magician, etc., are believed to be strongest

   (n.) A time when almost nobody has any reason to be out. These times usually occur at night but may happen at any time, depending on the day.

Lynn usually eats too many snacks during witching hour because no one is home and she is very hungry. Lynn has no self-control during witching hour, and neither do you.

#bored #noonehome #hungry #cantstopeating #stuffmyface

This witching hour is impossible to escape once you have entered. No human being has ever escaped this period if she has entered it hungry. No one has ever escaped under the mind-set that she plans on snlacking. Snlacking is what happens when you start having a snack. It then turns into a fiasco because you are unable to find what you are looking for. You start with something small. You keep eating and eating, trying to please that craving that you can't figure out you have. You are lacking self-control. You are lacking an actual idea of what you want. You are definitely lacking any willpower since the godforsaken gargoyles have taken over. They beat you again.

Snlacking

verb

snlacked; snlacking; snlacks

intransitive verb

1. to eat a snack without a plan

   (v.) Eating in small quantity but frequently and without a plan. This is done usually mindlessly without thought or calculation. To snack is to eat a small quantity of food between meals or instead of a main meal but lacking control or desire to have a plan or portion control.

   Gerald was snlacking after work, and he ate so much that he ruined his appetite and decided that he is a worthless pig. Gerald knows if he keeps snlacking that he will never get his weight under control and most likely never get laid or even kiss a girl.

   #nocontrol #lackasnack #noplan #bingemeal #poorGerald #stepawayfromthecookies

There is no point in discussing dinner or any other food choices until I teach you how to combat these demons and put them to rest. I have to warn you. These relentless assholes are invincible. The never die. They're like Freddie fuckin' Krueger who keeps coming back. Time after time and just when you think he's dead ... *bam* ... He slits your throat. Since we know we can't destroy them, we have to outsmart them. For as strong and powerful as their forces may be, they are pretty stupid. It doesn't take much to fool them, and if you do your job, they will go away and leave you alone as long as you keep your guard up. It's kind of like *Ghostbusters*. At three o'clock, you have to put your white suit and backpack on and get ready to take these monsters down so they don't take you down.

Gargoyles be gone ...

Now that you are aware of this dangerous time of day, I need to teach you the strategies that will are needed to get through it. Every damn day. Like anything, the most difficult part is starting. I had a difficult time with this. I had to visualize myself in full camo and war gear heading into the day at witching hour. My automatic rifle was ready to fire. What was I firing at? These invisible gargoyles who would destroy me every single day. Yep, I would shoot my imaginary rifle at these invisible creatures. They made me stuff my face every day at three o'clock when I had no control because I allowed myself to lack control.

You read that right. I would stand there with my pretend rifle in my fucking pretend combat boots waiting to shoot these pretend assholes who made me snlack. Every day I was ready. Every day I would get outsmarted and lose to these monsters. Every day I would end up stuffing my face and ruining my dinner appetite, as well as my desire to ever want to diet again. Until one day I figured it out, accidentally.

Successful Snacking

The day the gargoyles died.

Ah ... what a day that was. I still remember the first one. As stupid as it sounds, I was either going to put duct tape on my mouth or have my dentist wire my jaw shut. If you think I am kidding, ask my kid brother. I persuaded him to go through dental school just to learn how to wire mouths shut for weight loss reasons. He is now a very successful dentist, thanks to me and my brilliant ideas. He has only wired jaws shut that need repair ... and mine has never qualified.

Anyhow, since my nonconventional methods were unrealistic, I decided I needed to go old school. I was going to actually have a high protein snack at two thirty, even though I wasn't hungry. You see, I always viewed this two thirty snack as a waste of calories. I mean, I had just had lunch a few hours ago for God's sake. Why was I forcing myself to eat again when I wasn't even hungry?? Then I did some math. I'm going to share a little story with you. Let's see how many of you can relate.

Gabrielle had a healthy breakfast and lunch. Her calories were exactly on point. She was feeling good about her food decisions for the day and was not at all hungry for a snack. Gabrielle had been on this health kick, so she had packed her Greek yogurt and almonds. This snack totals 180 calories and almost 20 grams of protein. She loved her midday yogurt snack. In her head, Gabrielle was also thinking she would like to save the 180 calories. She could have an extra glass of wine or piece of chocolate after dinner.

Time ticked away, and now it was closer to three thirty. Gabrielle was feeling a little hungry, but also thought having her snack now was counterproductive. Dinner was in a few hours. Gabrielle was still okay with the decision to not eat her yogurt because she was not starving. She knew that her glass of wine or chocolate would be worth it.

It was four o'clock, and the hunger pains had started. Gabrielle decided to eat the almonds to tide her over since they wouldn't be that bad. She pulled out the jar of almonds. Instead of measuring out the ten almonds that she was supposed to have with her yogurt, she had a few handfuls—not that many, though … (Little did Gabrielle know that the gargoyles had taken over. They were perched on her shoulder. They had a food scale and calculator and were keeping track of calories consumed in her midday splurge).

The almonds did the trick.

They sure did … They got Gabrielle's taste buds going, and now she was really craving something sweet.

She decided that she was going to have her piece of post-dinner chocolate now. She told herself that she had already earned it, and then she wouldn't want anything else.

Gabrielle was very confident that this would work.

She was thrilled.

She was going to be smart and have some baby carrots while she made dinner.

Great idea, she thought ... until she realized her jaw was like the motor of a Vitamix. *It's okay*, she thought. *They're just carrots*. She told herself she wouldn't eat as much dinner.

Meanwhile, the gargoyles were calculating those calories on their little calculators. They high-fived each other on another successful mission.

Dinnertime ... Because Gabrielle's snacks from three thirty until now had virtually no protein, she was hungry after all. She ended up eating dinner despite the fact that she thought she wouldn't need to. She had her wine and, of course, another piece of chocolate. Disappointed that she had that second piece of chocolate, she capped off the night with a cookie and called it a day. In the end, Gabrielle knew she didn't have the best day, but she didn't think she did terrible.

Let's see what the Gargoyles calculated as calories mindlessly eaten.

+ A few handfuls of almonds in reality was 2 ounces, equaling 360 calories
+ Chocolate square that was to be for after dinner, 110 calories
+ Baby carrots at 5 calories each, 150 calories (plus the ranch she didn't mention), 300 calories
+ The wine that she had because she didn't have the yogurt, 150 calories

+ The chocolate she had again because she was mad that she had the chocolate already, 150 calories

+ The cookie she had because she was mad that she had the chocolate, 350 calories

+ Total: 1,570 extra calories

Are you yanking my chain? What kind of cruel joke is this? Gabrielle didn't even eat anything that bad.

Right?!

For the love of God, people, do you see here why it is so hard to lose weight?!

The woman ate almonds and baby carrots for fuck's sake.

Okay, she had some chocolate. The thought of her having 1,570 extra calories in crap ... Keep in mind that she did this mindlessly because she wasn't hungry at 2:30. Mind-boggling!

Listen here, people.

I realize her little frickin' cup of Greek yogurt may not have saved the day. She should have eaten it at snack time with her ten almonds. This combination of high protein and healthy fat would have kept the gargoyles away. Gabrielle would not have eaten 2 ounces of almonds, which is not too much but equals 360 calories. This set off the afternoon binge that cost her more than a thousand calories and her sanity.

Keep in mind she had 1,570 calories not including her breakfast, lunch, dinner, and morning snack. She stayed spot on for these meals. This made it that much more disheartening in the end when Gabrielle evaluated her intake for the day. She thought she did well. Meanwhile, the scale isn't moving, and Gabrielle is getting fluckstrated. So I ask you, would it have been better for her to have her 180-calorie snack instead of snlacking all afternoon?

Gargoyles be gone …

So how did I combat this? How did I destroy these little fuckers who would torture me every damn day? They would make me lose control by fogging my brain with the inability to make logical food choices. I swear it was like watching myself be taken away by the body snatchers every flipping day. Every day these monsters would come and spray something through the air. This would make me suddenly forget what calories even were. It was like laughing gas for people who need to gain weight. You breathe this shit, and you have to put every edible thing in your mouth. Everything, whether it tastes good or not, and chew it. How the fuck do you combat this?

One day, I was in my kitchen inhaling this appetite-inducing laughing gas. I had to make these *healthy* snacks for my daughter's class. My famous *peanut butter balls.* Are you wondering why I emphasized the word *healthy*? It's because the ingredients consist of all nutritious things: peanut butter, honey, oats, chia seeds, flax seeds, raisins, cinnamon, almond butter, craisins, and sunflower seeds. Delicious!

Yes, but if you look at the gargoyle's calculator, they are about 150 calories each. Each one is only the size of a golf ball. Who has time to worry about that when it's witching hour and the Gargoyles are under watch? I'm not implying that you shouldn't make these, but if you do, they are fucking orgasmic. You mix everything together and make them into little meatball-sized love nuggets. They are healthy, but you shouldn't eat fifteen of them like I did that day. Okay, if you counted the mouthfuls of batter I shoveled in, it may have been more like nineteen. My point is that I was pretty full— full of an extra 2,280 calories of peanut butter, oats, and flax seeds. Let me take a quick moment to explain to you all what happens to raw oatmeal and flaxseeds when they get wet.

They expand. Throw in some chia seeds and peanut butter, and you pretty much don't need to eat ever again.

That's right, my friends, the laughing gas I was breathing caused me to inhale a catastrophic amount of gut-binding ingredients. I could have pretty much lived on a deserted island for at least forever. The bad part is, my brain wasn't able to comprehend how full I was until it was far too late. Now keep in mind that these peanut butter balls were healthy. Since I didn't measure or count what I had sucked down, I had no idea that I had consumed 2,280 calories. In addition, I'd consumed 152 grams of fat (true story). In my head, I was thinking I didn't do much damage, and I was prepared to eat dinner a few hours later. Wrong.

Super wrong.

Super-duper, insanely wrong …

As I prepared dinner that evening, I noticed that there was a lot less finger lickin' going on. The normal bites and nibbles of each ingredient didn't seem appealing to me. The crazy thing is I actually noticed the absence of my usual sampling. I rinsed my fingers off in the sink instead of in my mouth. It's like I noticed, but I stashed that information in the denial part of my brain. Admitting that I noticed meant I would have to stop denying that I ate half of my dinner while making my dinner. I would have to stop denying that I would eat another full portion during dinner. My point is that I was so full from making a pig out of myself that I was unable to make a pig out of myself.

Later that afternoon the kids got home from school, bringing the usual chaos along with them. First, they need a snack, and then they need to be taken to activities. Exhausted, I got them all home and got dinner on the table. As I prepared plates for each of my little monsters like the slave-mother that I have become, I realized that I didn't dive into their afterschool snack. I didn't eat most of their post-activity treat, and I didn't eat part of their dinner serving their dinner. While I sat down and watched them all not eat the dinner I had lovingly prepared, I realized why I had not eaten the usual astronomical number of calories during the witching hour. The gargoyles were sitting on my shoulder with their calculators.

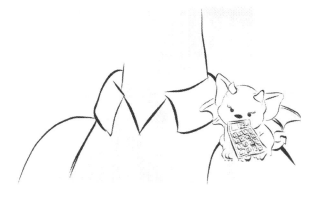

They were waiting to enter in the damaging amounts of calories consumed during this witching hour until dinner. Nothing.

This got me thinking. The key was to be full enough from three o'clock until dinner to avoid my brain being captured by the gargoyles. I needed to do this again, but I needed to figure out a way to do it without consuming a half a million calories and making a pig of myself. *Bingo!* My epiphany. I used my knowledge as a nutritional coach and my experience as an individual who has failed at every diet ever and created the *binge blocker*.

Binge Blocker

(n.) A small snack that contains high levels of protein and healthy fat that should be eaten before a meal. This snack is to help prevent overeating or binging. Binge blockers should contain 20 grams of protein and 10 grams of fat and should not exceed 300 calories.

I am a fucking genius!

For real, if you haven't figured this out yet, I am a goddamn fucking genius.

Eat before you eat, and then you won't want to eat!

What the fuck, people?!

It's not hard!

I realize that there are snacks you can have, but a regular snack won't do jack shit. Some crackers, cheese, or fruit are a teasers.

Give me a break.

Those one-hundred-calorie packs are nothing but a good way to pollute the earth with more trash.

Now we have to open ten of these fuckers to be satisfied instead of one big bag.

I also get to pay extra to do so.

To top it off, these snacks have nowhere near enough protein and fat to satisfy your hunger. The goal is to feel *peanut butter ball full* without the 2,280 calories and 152 grams of fat. It's possible. I spent the next few days experimenting. I created several binge blockers that fit this profile and were very satisfying. Make sure you bookmark this page. Start including these gargoyle-repelling treats in your daily routine. I also suggest you have one of these binge blockers before going out to eat. Eat one before going to a party. Have one before attending any situation where the gargoyles may make an appearance.

Gargoyles be gone …

Binge Blockers

Keep portions moderate (snack size). The purpose for these is to keep you full and stabilize your insulin levels, which will keep you from binging.

My top picks:

Most of these are less than 300 calories and more than 20 grams of protein and 10 grams of *healthy* fat, which will keep you full.

- 1 can of tuna or 3 ounces chicken and 1/2 avocado or 2 tablespoons hummus
- 1 cup of cottage cheese or Greek yogurt with 10 almonds or 1 tablespoon of peanut butter
- 2 hard-boiled eggs
- a protein shake with 1 tablespoon of peanut butter

These are meant to be snacks, not meals. Don't add veggies or add-ins, so they're quick and you won't *feel* full. Often, the full feeling triggers more eating.

Once I started incorporating these snacks into my day, I lost 20 pounds, but I was also able to repair my metabolism. Your body wants to be fed and nourished every few hours. Don't deprive it, and it will treat you well.

I also feel very compelled so share my famous *peanut butter ball* recipe with you. Eat these treats with caution, and for the *love of God*, have a binge blocker before you make them.

Getufit Peanut Butter Balls

6 cups raw old-fashioned oatmeal

2 cups peanut butter

1 cup almond butter

1 cup honey

1/2 cup chia seeds

1 cup whole flaxseeds

1 cup raisins

1/2 cup craisins

1/2 cup sunflower seeds

1 tablespoon cinnamon

Mix ingredients. With wet hands, form golf ball–sized (or smaller) balls. This should make several dozen peanut butter bites. Eat with caution. *They are high in calories.*

9

Self-Sabotage:
The Wrecking Ball

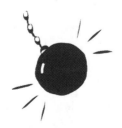

I don't understand why, but the practice of self-massacre is not only common but has been in practice for years.

People like to take themselves down. People wait until they are at the peak of success. Then they sit back and watch a wrecking ball rip everything apart. The problem here is that the wrecking ball is being controlled by you.

Like Miley Cyrus sang in her 2013 hit song, "I came in like a wrecking ball … I just closed my eyes and swung …"

Anyone who has ever destroyed her own progress has come in with this wrecking ball. Come in full-steam ready to destroy. Often, this demolition is unplanned. Sometimes this attack comes with a faint premonition of it coming, almost like an aura. It might be a bright light or sensation. It's something that comes about you that is telling you to go rage on your food plan. Suddenly, you are planning to extinguish every bit of work you have put forth on this diet. When you hear a demonic voice grumbling inside your head telling you that this game is over, you know the wrecking ball is coming.

Why?

Why would we work so hard on something to sit back and watch ourselves destroy it? It's such an unexplainable phenomenon. People do it all the time with all aspects of life, but with health and wellness, I am particularly intrigued. Why would someone spend weeks or months working so hard only to destroy it? Change her eating and lifestyle to take it down with one clean sweep? This behavior has always made me want to study the depths of the human psyche and why the human brain would allow such destruction to take place. A person who has devoted so much time, energy, and money to a cause shouldn't want to ruin things. So why does it happen?

As I mentioned earlier in this book, unless you find a sustainable plan, you only have a 5 percent chance of keeping weight off that you lose. That's it. There are many reasons for this. These reasons are covered throughout this book, the top one being this wrecking ball. It has a 95 percent likelihood of swinging your way during this bumpy ride. If you know it's coming, you can protect yourself and avoid getting hit.

Let's pull up our Wonder Woman underpants, girls. I'm going to teach you how to avoid this self-sabotage. What is self-sabotage? I have been telling my self-sabotaging clients this story for years. It's about an artist who spent many, many months working on a very detailed project.

The Beautiful Wall

Matteo was an artist who had a passion for detail. One day he decided he wanted to paint a mural for himself as an expression of his love for art. This mural was the size of a large room and had a multitude of colors. Every day Matteo would go to his old warehouse that he rented. He had this room that he spent hours planning, prepping, and preparing for the next steps in the process. He used very detailed tools to apply all the different colors of paint. He also spent hours shopping for this paint so the colors would be perfect. He waited for the paint to dry before moving on to the next step in order for everything to be ideal. Every single day Matteo could see his progress on the walls of this mural. Anyone who had seen his work praised him for his dedication and commitment.

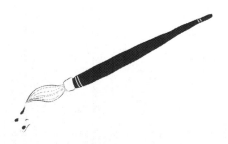

One thing about Matteo was that he had never completed a project such as this before, and he was starting to get a bit nervous that at some point he was going to do something to mess things up. In fact, he started to feel anxious about the mural and found himself going to the warehouse less often. He also found that he wasn't enjoying it as much but couldn't figure out why. This scared him a bit, so he figured he needed to take a break. Matteo talked himself into this well-deserved break and decided to go back to do a little painting again. To his sad surprise, it wasn't the same. He couldn't get into it. This made Matteo sad and even more anxious. He decided to leave and take an entire week off to clear his head and figure out a new plan.

During this time off, Matteo thought about his mural and all his months of hard work. He was reminded of how much he missed it. He was thrilled at his newly sparked enthusiasm and headed back to the warehouse to paint. Super excited to get there and get started, he discovered that he never properly cleaned up the last time he was there, and as a result, the brushes were all ruined. Disappointed, yet not discouraged, he would run to the craft store and treat himself to some new brushes and paints. *That's what women do, right?* he thought as he filled his cart. A new set of forty-eight premium artist brushes, an acrylic paint kit with seventy-one colors, an aluminum easel, and a glaze kit. He felt reborn. New supplies, new inspiration. He headed back to the warehouse to paint but decided to set everything up and come back when he had more time.

Weeks had passed now. The new supplies had been sitting at the studio untouched. Matteo has been unmotivated and absent from this project that he once cared so much about. He felt it coming … He sensed this feeling of "I don't know what," as he explained it. Frustrated, he went to the warehouse and decided to work. He needed to get back on track. New brushes, new paint. He dipped, stroked, painted, sketched, shaped, doodled, scribbled, scratched, screeched, and screamed ... He kept going. Scribbling, smearing, scarring, and now defacing his work. He thought he was getting on track, but his frustrations led him to destroy his work. Without realizing it, Matteo had taken black paint and painted over all the beautiful details— the details that he had worked so hard to create. Months and months of work. Days and hours of planning and prepping. Gone. He had completely sabotaged his project and destroyed it. What he had worked so hard to accomplish was ruined. Matteo even had a premonition that this self-mutilating behavior was on the horizon. This had happened many times before. He was so close to finishing, yet still so far.

You can see that this artist is no different than we are. Matteo painting black paint over his work is no different than jumping into the bowl of guacamole at a party. Anyone who has ever lost weight has spent countless hours planning and prepping for her success.

It is not a part-time thing. It is a 24/7 deal. There is not a minute that doesn't go by when a food decision doesn't have to be made. We are faced with hundreds of food decisions every day. Day in, day out. Every week. For every month. For however long you make it before that wrecking ball gets wheeled out. It presents itself like the next fucking game on the *Price Is Right*. "Matteo, you are the next contestant in the *Price Is Right!*" You hear that, and you're screwed. The wrecking ball is out. Up until now you have always surrendered to your weaknesses and let it take you down. Not this time. Where are those Wonder Woman undies? Pull those fuckers up. I have to teach you a few things about avoiding self-sabotage.

Avoiding Self-Sabotage

Set realistic, sustainable goals. Be real. As I mentioned earlier, don't set your goals so high that they are not sustainable. You have to be mindful of the fact that you need to be able to continue this routine for a long time. How long, you ask? Um … forever. Don't be an ass. If you can't hold your breath for five minutes, then you should not take the chance of diving too deep and drowning. Pick a more realistic time limit. Sabotaging weight-loss efforts involves more than cheating on your diet. It happens when you set goals you can't meet.

Go the distance. Your goal is to lose weight and see an immediate result. Cutting in line and cheating will only slow you down. Instead of moving fast, take small, realistic steps toward your goal. It may take longer to reach your goal, but you will most likely stick to your plan. As you become accustomed to the changes involved, you could add more intensity to your program. Add changes as tolerated instead of all at the beginning. This is when you are overwhelmed and most likely to quit. For example, add one more day of exercise to your week and stick to it for a month. Add one more glass of water to your daily intake over the course of the week. This way, you're not choking down dozens of ounces at once. Change your nutritional routine gradually. Don't wipe your cupboards of all foods at once. Making everyone in your family eat kale and quinoa exclusively for a week straight may not be the best idea. Eventually, you may truly love your kale and quinoa. But don't force it down all day and end up eating a greasy cheeseburger for dinner. Then you didn't go the distance. There are plenty of people who become accustomed to such healthy and clean diets. They could tell you that it was a transition. Your pallet will adjust to the new textures, flavors, and varieties of foods. They will become your new favorites. Be sure to allow room for some of your classic favorites—with moderation, of course. No marathon runner ever got a medal for running twenty-five miles. It's that last stretch that counts. Set yourself up for success!

Hold the pose. Once you create a routine that you like, you have to decide if you can sustain that routine for a long time or permanently. As you are going through the motions of the new regimen, you will have yourself convinced that you love it. You will think that you can undoubtably do it forever. When weight loss occurs, you experience a bit of euphoria. This causes your brain to think you can maintain certain routines than may not be realistic. I have seen this happen. I have seen this happen hundreds of times over the years. People either restrict their calories to low levels, causing rapid weight loss, or spend hours a day at the gym. These diet cheaters will inevitably end up getting caught cheating or cutting in line. This will lead to the wrecking ball making its appearance and striking once again. You have to dig deep into your psyche. It is difficult to identify the differences between realistic and unsustainable. When you find yourself cutting too many corners and taking those shortcuts, you have to dial things back and make an important decision. Choosing to continue on with an unsustainable routine will bring you faster results, but these results will inevitably be temporary. Being realistic may make the weight take longer to come off, but you will be happier during the process. As a result, your chances of keeping it off will increase substantially. Be very conscientious about these things as your program develops, and keep it real.

Face your fears. You always have the best intentions the day before. People always plan on going to the gym the next day. We always intend to follow that food plan and avoid the temptations of the world. We spend countless hours planning and playing the imaginary scripts of the perfect day in our heads every single day—until the day actually comes. After you have promised yourself that you would go to the gym at seven o'clock that morning, a friend calls for breakfast. Or you're running late for work. Or you're too tired to get up that early. Then you convince yourself that you will go tomorrow for sure, and the cycle of procrastination continues. Procrastination. Procrastination. Procrastination. *Procrastination.* No matter how you read it, it all spells the same thing: *avoidance.* If you wanted to get up and go to the gym at seven o'clock, nothing would stop you. Nothing. If this seven o'clock meeting was a job interview or a hair appointment, you would never ever miss it. What does this tell you? The likely culprit in this situation is fear. To start a new course, you must ask yourself, "Why am I afraid to go to the gym?" Believe it or not, gym-a-phobia is a true thing. I suffered from it and still do sometimes. Can there be anything more intimidating than walking into a fully loaded gym? Now walk in when you already don't feel like a superstar. Or maybe you feel fine with the gym environment but feel week or view yourself like a failure. Perhaps you want to save yourself the embarrassment of not knowing how to use the treadmill. Maybe you don't even where to hang your coat. You need to figure out what you are afraid of. There is a reason why you aren't allowing yourself to succeed. Until you figure it out, that wrecking ball may strike. Following are some common reasons that people fear success.

Being afraid of success. What will life be like after weight loss? Often people fear the unknown. This irrational fear of not knowing what life will be like after losing a tremendous amount of weight can be scary for some people. Being unable to comprehend weighing dozens of pounds less could scare someone enough to cause them to avoid it.

Keeping the weight off. There is a lot of stress involved in maintaining the routine involved. Knowing the amount of work involved, people fear the realization of having to maintain the same habits for the rest of their lives. Understanding that the new program should be realistic should help with the sustainability of the routine.

Fearing failure. Many are afraid that starting a program will lead to another unsuccessful attempt. Many times, individuals have failed several times prior in similar programs. This fear of repeating their failure is one that may prevent them from making another attempt.

Battling self-doubt. People often have low self-esteem and struggle with the ability to perceive themselves succeeding. Until people have succeeded in something, they may feel uneasy about their ability to perform the tasks necessary to meet their goals.

<u>Losing that safety blanket</u>. The weight presents itself as a safety blanket that protects you from taking action in intimidating situations. Losing this blanket will cause great fears.

<u>Fearing lifestyle change</u>. Losing weight may lead to dating, expanding your social life, having to maintain daily exercise, or having to shop for new clothes and understand fashion. All of these things are irrational yet relevant fears.

<u>Fearing negative priority changes</u>. You may worry that weight loss might cause you to take time away from your family due to more time at the gym or food prepping.

<u>Fearing judgement</u>. People will cast judgement upon others for anything and everything. Having a fear of others judging you for why you lost weight or why you needed to lose weight is a legitimate obstacle.These are headings and should be underlined

<u>Stop comparing yourself to others</u>. We live in a hypercompetitive society. We have become a nation of individuals who batter and bruise the egos of others. All in the same breath, we compare ourselves to everyone else and measure ourselves based on other people's standards. It is essential to avoid comparing ourselves to our peers. This competition can become unhealthy and counterproductive.

Every person is completely different. We all have different metabolic rates. We all move at different rates and at different levels throughout the day. Furthermore, we all eat and drink different foods. Our bodies respond to this nutrition in a variety of different ways. There is no way you can take one person's routine and expect it to work on someone else. You also can't expect to achieve the same results as another individual. You think that person may be following the same plan as you, but in reality, that is impossible. In addition to you comparing your progress to that of others, you also assume you are following the same plan. This is where social media can be dangerous. It can be depressing to go on someone's Instacrap account and see a nonstop flow of overdone gym look-at-me selfies. These pictures are screaming low self-esteem from every post. I can tell you that Wendy the Workout Queen is not following the same plan as you. Her plan is called *a camera filter*. It's one that makes her ass look rounder and her waist look smaller. The chances that she is on the same plan as you are slim to none. Even if the plans were similar, you should not compare your progress to that of others. These constant calculations and comparisons will cause an unnecessary amount of stress and anxiety in your life. It will do you no good. Be your own person, and praise yourself for your progress. Wendy is stupid anyway, and I heard she's had work done … #imontoyouWendy #bewhoyouare

Challenge yourself. Don't be afraid of taking risks. It is always easy to settle into a routine that is comfortable, especially when you have experienced success with something. The most successful people are always pushing limits and expanding boundaries. Past triumphs are important. Those victories can equip you with the confidence you need to achieve your current goals. If you're spending too much time celebrating your old successes, you're not challenging yourself enough. This is necessary to meet new goals. Don't be afraid of failure. Sometimes taking risks means that you are going to fall on your ass. That fall is one that is usually worth taking. Although you may lose some skin on the fall, you will most likely learn some things. These things will help you grow and do new things. Individuals who self-sabotage often hold themselves back. They don't give themselves enough credit for having the ability to take these risks.

Always learn from a good mistake. I have never taken a bad mistake and not learned something good from it. There is a silver lining around every dark cloud. You just have to find it. Don't be so hard on yourself as you work toward your goals. There is *no way* you will get through any process without making a mistake. No matter how organized or brilliant you think you are, you will make a mistake. First off, you have to learn how to self-forgive. This is a biggie. Don't beat yourself up for past lapses in judgement. Don't let your mind torment you. Tune out all negativity, and think about how you could have made the situation better. Learn from the mistake and move on.

As you can see from reading this chapter, it is human nature to sabotage ourselves for many things. When it comes to weight loss, this is extremely common. As I have worked with people over the years, I have come to the realization that this is an expected part of the process. It is probable that almost every person I have worked with comes to a point in the program when they feel the need to sabotage themselves. This was going to inevitably occur, so I decided to start telling my clients that this was going to happen. I was hoping that telling them would deter the behavior. I found that knowing that this behavior may occur reduced the likelihood of it happening. Being aware of the strategies that could be taken will keep the *wrecking ball* at bay. There is a fine line between those who welcome the wrecking ball to demolish their hard work and those who do not want that ball to harm them. I am going to share two similar stories of two individuals.

It is clear who has invited the wrecking ball into her life and who does not want the ball to strike.

Avanna and Samantha have been best friends since they can remember and do everything together. When Avanna decided to get highlights, Samantha would also get highlights. If the highlights were hot pink, then hot pick it was for both. When Samantha wanted to learn sign language, Avanna also signed up for the class. When Avanna wanted to go rock climbing, Samantha gave her best attempt. Monkey see, monkey do.

Although they did everything together, the two of them were quite opposite in nature. Avanna was not very organized and was often impulsive, whereas Samantha was generally over-the-top with her to-do lists and plans. These besties were so opposite that it was a constant joke. If one of them was cold, the other was hot ... but they were probably wearing the same outfit and eating the same thing.

Their eating patterns were not so good at all. Fast-food junkies, followed by processed meals with low nutritional quality, topped off with foods containing high preservatives. They were like two happy clams sitting in their apartment ordering crappy food. Night after night, they ate guiltlessly with not a worry in the world. As the two of them gained weight, they both planned to get their poor eating habits under control. They knew they would do it together ... of course. After one weekend full of Chinese food and a sushi spread large enough to feed all Japan, they decided it was time. One last celebration. They would make these amazing pretzel and peanut butter Rolo cookies and eat them right out of the oven, and they were ready to diet.

Samantha spent all day and part of the night reorganizing the cabinets and labeling everything. Avanna finished watching season 12 of *Hollywood Firefighter Wives*. They decided they were going to figure out which food plan was best for them. Samantha had spent endless hours researching and could probably already write a book about weight loss. Avanna was too busy worrying about what Netflix series she was going to binge next. They selected the plan that Samantha picked.

Let me give you some background on these two ladies. Samantha was very type A, as you already know. All her i's were dotted, and her t's were always crossed. Her i's were even dotted with fucking hearts. Even now. She's Mrs. Happy Pants 100 percent of the time, and to top it off, she teaches kindergarten. Fucking kindergarten. Let's be real! In the event that I might be that goddamn happy, there would for sure be alcohol involved. The second a five-year-old would make themselves present with their mousy little voice, I would lose my happy pants and my shit all at once. Yep, happy pants and shit all in one nice little bundle.

That would be me, and that was exactly Avanna most of the time. For as perky and annoying—I mean, enthusiastic—as Samantha could be, her BFF was less than pleasant. I wouldn't say Avanna was mean or vicious, but let's just say she filled with a lot less perk and a lot more jerk.

Both of these ladies had a tremendous amount of friends. Their friends were of completely different cultures. It was like the Pink Ladies versus the Women of Wrestling. It didn't matter because Sam and Alex were good for each other, even though their friends had legal restraining orders against one another. The reason I tell you this is because I think it's fucking hysterical, yet has nothing to do with the story or them. Anyhow, back to the diet ...

> Their new lifestyle started off a bit bumpy but went well overall. Samantha would cook everything and prep. Avanna would complain that she didn't like certain things. Then she would end up loving everything she tried. Samantha would enter every meal perfectly calculated into her log. Avanna

would just ask her for the information and throw it in all at the end of the day. Avanna would weigh herself every morning and record her weight. Samantha would wait until after she exercised to get a fake weight and then enter it into her log. She would then cry on Avanna's shoulder that she was getting tired of this routine.

They kept going. Samantha would set her alarm every day and force herself out of bed. Avanna would get up only when she felt like it. Samantha would get super stressed if she forgot to pack a lunch and spend her lunch hour trying to figure out what to eat. Avanna would also forget but make appropriate choices. Day in, day out ... week after week ... month after month. These two ladies battled out all the quarrels that occur with yourself when you are losing weight. At this point, both of these ladies had hit plateaus and had been able to move on. They had both lost more than thirty pounds and were feeling great, yet losing momentum.

One day Samantha felt herself really slipping. She couldn't describe it, but she felt like she was getting tired of maintaining this routine—the logging, cooking, shopping, prepping, and working out. She was super tired of doing everything for Avanna. It was double the work. To make things worse, she felt like she would be letting Avanna down if she quit or took a break. This terrible pressure that she felt spiraled into more anxiety.

Samantha was feeling like not only could she not maintain this routine, but she felt she was not going to be able to keep the weight off, thus making her a failure. She thought back to the last time she lost thirty-three pounds. The same thing happened. She became derailed and ended up gaining back all her weight. She had such a fear of being judged again, and with her type A personality, that just can't happen. No way, no how. Miss Perfect Pants couldn't fail at anything, and if this was a fail, then she was a fail. Perfect Pants and Happy Pants go together. There is no room for Self-Doubt Pants, and she would rather have fat pants in her closet than look-at-me-I-failed pants.

As crazy as it sounds, Samantha basically opened the door and invited the gargoyles in. She walked up to her brain and opened the doors. She invited all elements self-doubt, uncertainty, and disbelief in. She let mistrust, paranoia, skepticism, and self-pity into her soul. These emotions, all in the physical presence of gargoyles, scurried up her body. They went into her head like the scrubbing bubbles in the bathroom cleaner commercials.

Once these fuckers are released, they saturate your mind, body, and soul. You remember the gargoyles? Those relentless little motherfuckers. They have this insane ability to cause your brain to do illogical things. In this case, when you open the pity party gates, these gargoyles like to *party*. They even throw confetti around. This causes you to have feelings of self-doubt and uncertainty. Like any confetti, this self-doubt confetti is a bitch to clean up.

> Samantha thought she wouldn't be able to maintain this new lifestyle days ago, so she had no desire to even try. She had convinced herself that it was too difficult and that she didn't have time. As time passed, Samantha came up with more and more reasons for why she didn't need to continue with this lifestyle. What she was actually doing was watching the wrecking ball demolish all her hard work. Every time that wrecking ball swung, those Gargoyles would cheer. They cheered as they shoved buttered popcorn down their conniving throats. Samantha did nothing to stop this. Strike after strike, the gargoyles celebrated this victory. Samantha

allowed this self-sabotaging behavior to take control once again.

On the other hand, Avanna had a bit less of an uptight attitude about certain things. Actually, she wasn't uptight about anything. She didn't give a rat's ass about what anyone thought about her or her lowlife idiot friends. Avanna was clearly a train wreck— the kind that Jerry Springer loves to have on his live panel when he's not revealing DNA who's-your-daddy results. Yet, Avanna was content with herself and her choices in life. She did nothing to please anyone else. If she set out to do anything, it was for herself and herself only.

Like I said, Avanna did not give a fuck about what anyone thought. If she went down in failure flames, she had no qualms about wearing that on her sleeve. She was a badass, and badasses don't cry. After she watched her bestie light her weight-loss-success pants on fire, she wondered if she would end up falling into that same rut.

So far, Avanna was feeling pretty confident about her weight loss and routine. She didn't allow herself to get overwhelmed by taking on too much with this new program. Although she followed the same plan as Samantha, she learned from her mistakes. She forgave herself for not being perfect. Unlike Miss Happy Pants, Avanna knew there was no such thing as perfect—except, of course, Lily Lankwather from season 6 of *Hollywood Firefighter Wives*. That girl had her shit together and was truly perfect ... but anyhow, no one else was perfect, and Avanna knew that. Things became more difficult now that Samantha wasn't on board with the clean eating. She had to pick up the slack for herself and actually prepare her own meals and cook for herself. Every so often she would stumble and make terrible mistakes that would result in small setbacks. She always self-forgave and learned from each mistake. Every time Avanna felt those gargoyles knocking, she avoided the temptations. When she felt the wrecking ball starting to swing, she would persevere with her positive attitude.

She was not doing this for others. She was doing this for herself. She liked eating these foods. She liked feeling this way. She enjoyed the energy that came with the weight loss and the clarity she felt with her newly found self-esteem. No matter what, she was not going to let that wrecking ball strike. She knew she was in control. Ultimately, she was able to avoid any self-sabotaging behaviors, which would eventually lead to her success.

Looking at the two stories, you can see how one of the characters allowed the negativity and self-sabotaging behaviors. It is my belief that Samantha was tired of the program. She didn't enjoy it anymore, and she was overwhelmed with the amount of work that it had become. She also created this extremely high expectation for herself to succeed with no room for errors. Her standards were set so high, and she had broadcast them to the world and felt somewhat trapped. Samantha realized she could no longer maintain this lifestyle. Instead of quitting or failing, she created obstacles to make it impossible for her to succeed. Once she stumbled a little bit, she wasn't able to self-forgive. This led to a snowball effect of stumbles, which then led to the presentation of the wrecking ball.

You see, Samantha was in control the entire time. She could have managed this entire ordeal differently. This would have changed the outcome of her story. Changing her type A personality and overzealous ability to complicate things was unrealistic. Samantha could learn to make many improvements that would help her in the future. Due to her diligence, you would think that Samantha would been more successful. In this case, and often in many cases, this desire to be perfect can lead to failure.

Samantha allowed the wrecking ball to strike by inviting self-sabotage into her life. She did this simply by being unrealistic. She set her standards too high and made her goals unreachable. Her routine was too difficult to follow, and she created her own anxieties by not allowing for any errors. In addition to this, Samantha had no tolerance for mistakes. She was unable to forgive herself for making them. She could never learn from them. In the end, this did her a huge injustice.

Avanna, on the other hand, would take the opportunity to learn from every mistake. For example, when she would forget her lunch, she would make the effort to plan better in the future. This would help her have a backup plan for where she could go to get a lunch. Her BFF would spend her entire lunch hour beating herself up. She spent more time thinking about what a failure she thought she was. Sadly, these pity parties would end up with a food binge of some sort. Samantha also has a clear issue with facing her fears. She was afraid of failing, she was afraid of not being the best, and she was afraid of what everyone else would think of her. These fears were costing her success on so many levels. These fears were keeping her from taking risks. Being a risk-taker may end up in failure, and now we are back to where we started.

Avanna, with her I-don't-give-a-shit attitude, actually did give a shit. She just did not care what others think. She was okay with taking things slow. She was fine with going the distance and making small changes along the way. She was never a fan of going bat shit crazy and changing things all at once. Baby steps were her way ... who needed tyrannosaurus rex steps? She was okay with working out three days a week instead of seven. She didn't think she needed to put all her salads in fuckling mason jars every Sunday afternoon. She didn't need to label them with different color scrapbook paper. She also found no point in creating spreadsheets of ounces of water she drank or spreadsheets with exact times that she took a frickin' dump.

Avanna just did her thing. She ate when she was hungry. She logged her food without getting out a petri dish. She didn't need a microscope to get the exact micrograms of nutrients. She drank her water and made sure she was pooping. There was no need to weigh her poop—I mean, come on ... (Oops, I wasn't supposed to share that.) Basically, Avanna knew how to make this new style of living one that she was comfortable with. She also knew that no one would judge her for not being perfect, and she always self-forgave. This ability to forgive herself was critical in her success, and it will be in yours. It is an attribute that is inborn but can be learned as well.

Sabotaging yourself is a common and interesting phenomenon. We do it with many aspects of our lives. People sabotage their careers, their families, and their finances. Individuals sabotage their freedom, dignity, and even reputation for reasons that are unknown. The wrecking balls sit idle in everyone's psyches. We just have to learn how to keep them from striking.

10

Forgive Yourself: Kiss and Make Up

W hy are we so hard on ourselves? Seriously. Let's think about this. No other living being tortures themselves like the humans do.

Does the mama bear drown herself in self-pity when she isn't able to gather enough fish for her baby cubs to eat for the day? No. She just sucks it up and makes the little fuckers share what she has brought home and deal with it.

What about the neighborhood skunk? Do you think he gets all pissed off at himself for not spraying the asshole dog that keeps barking at them for no reason? No. The skunk moves on with his life and doesn't dwell on everything he should have done.

So why do we spend endless hours torturing ourselves? Just because we were unable to complete a certain task? Self-forgive, people! I really believe people have this desire to beat themselves to a pulp. We do this so that we can forget the real reason for why we are upset. I've had clients skip one workout and spend the entire day mad at themselves, so angry that it caused all sorts of negative behaviors. Poor eating choices and self-sabotaging behavior are at the top of the list.

How does this make sense? We all do it. We especially do it when it comes to food and eating. I've had clients eat perfectly all week—no glitches. But then, for some unexplained reason, they fall off the program and eat something that is not on the plan. It is important to realize that making mistakes is part of the process. It will happen from time to time. Instead, most people will let this destroy them. This will cause them to participate in more undesirable behaviors. The landslide of destruction will then lead to more disappointment in yourself. The vicious cycle begins. This can easily be fixed if you learn how to forgive yourself.

Let's say you were walking down the street and you bumped into a brick wall and smacked your head. Would you shake it off and move on, being careful not to bump your head again? Or would you pick up a brick off the ground to carry around with you so you could smack yourself in the head all day? If you said you would carry a brick around with you, then you are either full of shit or really fucked up and need professional help. You are not going to keep smacking yourself with a brick all day after you accidently hurt yourself. You're not. So, why is it that you will most likely punish yourself by eating an ungodly amount of shit after making one bad eating choice?

Lord knows I did this for years. Okay ... I did this for decades. I could write a book telling stories about my jacked-up food fiascos, but I guess that's what I am doing. I vividly remember a time when I was really struggling to maintain my weight. Every little variable would tip me off, and I was super sensitive to making sure I was spot on with the program. I was teaching school at the time. I had gained a bunch of weight the year before and finally had it under control by being on this new program. I was down eight pounds and feeling great. It was a Friday. The teachers had brought treats into the teachers' lounge to celebrate the weekend. We did this regularly to make sure everyone had enough calories shoved in their faces before starting the day. If that wasn't enough, there were bagels and cream cheese and fresh Danishes there as well.

Teachers love to eat. Teachers love to eat on Fridays. Teachers super love to make other teachers who are losing weight squirm. They want all dieters to cave and eat all the crap that is in the teachers' lounge. I resisted. I was a fucking rock star. I sat at my desk with my Snackwells zero-fat, no-sugar-added yogurt. I was loving how loose my pedal pushers were fitting. I adjusted my banana-clipped curly hair and ate my snack. Those fat fucks were not going to take me down.

The day progressed. I felt the donuts calling my name. For real, they were calling my name.

"Irene … You can hear us … Get your ass down here and just take half of one. You deserve it. Just half. You are doing so good, only a half a donut won't hurt you."

I know that you are reading this thinking I am crazy … but I also know you have been called to the kitchen by food yourself. Stop judging me, and keep reading my story.

"Irene … Irene … If you come take half a donut, we will leave you alone and stop bothering you."

Motherfucker, I thought. *These goddamn voices in my head again.*

I had made it through most of the day. I had a healthy lunch and stayed on the program all day, but the voices were back. Although it was feeding time, I knew I should have had my high-protein snack. I was once again summoned to the teachers' lounge. I knew I was in trouble. It was witching hour, and the gargoyles were waking from their nap. They were getting their calculators ready. The gargoyles like to use the old-school calculators with the paper tape. They love using this paper. It adds extra effect when it drapes over your shoulder as they enter in all the food you mindlessly throw down your throat.

I made the very conscious decision to go to the teachers' lounge and see for myself that there were probably no donuts left. After all, it was already two o'clock. I waited until my students were in PE class and dropped them off. The PE teacher was super hot, so I had to make sure I looked extra good before drop-off. That has nothing to do with the donuts or this book ... but it may come into play a little later. Anyhow, I then headed straight to the teachers' lounge. I noticed I was rushing there, as if I were in some sort of hurry.

Not understanding my rush, I got there to see that the donuts were pretty picked over. Luckily, there was enough of a selection for me to have the half a donut that I so desperately had been craving. There I stood. Me, myself, and the donuts—a few glazed, a maple, a Bavarian cream, a jelly filled, a few long Johns, and some frosted. They didn't look nearly as good as they did eight hours ago, but I knew I was only going to eat half of one, so I was okay with a little crustiness. The donuts sat in the grease-stained box all calling my name. They waved at me as if I were at an auction bidding for a priceless sculpture. I looked up the calories of each one so I could get the best deal for my splurge.

Bavarian cream has 550 calories? Fuck that shit. That's 225 for a half a donut. No way.

Jelly filled 350, glazed 200, long John 300, frosted 250, and I didn't look up the maple because who would eat that anyway? After much thought and consideration, I had made my decision. I was going with the long John. Although not the lowest in calories, I felt I was getting a little more for the splurge.

I was ready to attack ... plate, knife, napkin ... check ... check ... check ... I proceeded to cut the long John in half. Perfection. I sat down, looked at the tiny pillow of goodness, and took one bite.

Holy mother of God.

It was fucking amazing.

Seriously.

Not just a little good, but the kind of good that leads to a food-gasm.

You know what that is without me having to explain it. I now sat there having my food-gasm. The gargoyles rolled up their sleeves and got ready for a busy afternoon.

Initially, I was strong. I finished my 150-calorie food-gasm and regained my composure. It was almost time to get my students from PE class. Damn it. I had to face Mr. Perfection of Fitness. I'm sure *his* wife would never shove donuts down her throat when no one was looking. Disappointed in myself, I had to hurry because I had about ten minutes left to get things ready for the science experiment that we were working on. I headed back to my classroom. Sadly, the only thing on my mind was the other half of that donut.

"Ireeennnnnneeeeee …" I could actually hear it calling me.

No, for real. I could hear this fucking voice calling me into the teachers' lounge, literally begging me to eat the other half. At that point, I had legitimately talked myself into every possible reason to go back and eat the donut. Like a fucking zombie, I headed back to the teachers' lounge. I was walking like Eddie Munster, hoping to God that the remains of my long John would still be there.

Once I got to the lounge, I grabbed the other half of the long John, along with the Bavarian cream. I'm not quite sure what happened at the time, but my hand just reached out and took it. I ate the remains of the long John and wrapped the Bavarian cream in a napkin. I smuggled it back to my classroom. After all, if no one saw me eat it, it wouldn't count. At this point, I was not really mad at myself just yet. The long John was only 300 calories, and that's about what my afternoon cottage cheese snack was. I did have some uneasy feelings stirring in my gut about what my plans were with Mr. Bavarian Cream all nestled in my paperclip drawer. Only one hour left until dismissal, and then I would decide what I would do.

Looking back at this now, I can see that I planned on diving into the paperclip drawer all along. Why didn't I just eat the flipping donut right away? Why did I leave it there to torture myself with the decision of eating it or not when all along I planned on eating it? Why did I plan on eating it after I had eaten the long John? Yet, I had no intention of choosing it earlier when I was making a logical decision to enjoy a half a donut? I am pretty sure you can answer all these questions, and most of you reading this book have probably had very similar experiences. This all boils down to my inability to forgive myself for making a poor decision.

First off, the fact that I chose to have a half a donut is not a poor decision. It was not impulsive, it was planned out, it was well thought out, and it was truly something I wanted. I should have accepted that as a positive and enjoyed the 150-calorie treat. Instead, I spent the entire afternoon upset with myself for eating the donut. I then decided to make matters worse by punishing myself. This lack of self-forgiveness would have a long-lasting domino effect, as it would often carry into the next day, week, and even month. You see, I bumped my head on a wall and spent the rest of the day hitting myself with a brick.

There is this innate desire that we all have to be pleasers. We want to please others, but we also want to please ourselves. There are certain strategies to help you learn how to forgive yourself for the slips, hiccups, and mistakes. These fiascos will inevitably occur throughout this new way of living. Learning how to cope is essential to your success.

Strategies for Self-Forgiveness

Understand that it's done. Remind yourself that this act is now in the past, it is not present, and you are not currently doing it. Notice when the mind trap of blaming yourself for past events arises. See if you can acknowledge its presence and then remind yourself that you did make a mistake. Tell yourself that was the past, and you are going to learn from it. This practice of blaming does not support you or others in any way at all. Allow the process of forgiveness of this past event to surface. Begin to see it as something you can learn and grow from moving forward. This will free you up to be more skillful in the present.

Adapt a learning mind-set. We are always going to make mistakes in this life. Everyone does. But the key mind-set that turns this on its head and catalyzes growth and happiness is the learning mind-set. Every single experience in life contains information. This helps us get better and better with our intentions in life. You want to forgive yourself for a mistake that was made. Think about how you made the mistake, and determine what you could do different next time. Instead of being full of anger, take the mistake and learn from it. This will make each mistake a valuable resource and help you self-forgive all at the same time.

Understand that you are not alone. One of the first things to do is understand that you are not the first person who has made this mistake. It has likely been made thousands if not millions of times before you by other people. I am not condoning the action but simply letting you know that you are not alone. Many people have made this mistake in the face of common human challenges. One of the common things we do as humans is taking things personally to a fault. When we come to understand that no one is immune from being unskillful, we can begin to take it a little less personally. This helps us practice self-forgiveness.

Create a redo. Never underestimate the power of a redo. Write down how you would have done things if you could go back and do it again. In doing so, affirm that you learned from your past mistake. Remind yourself that if you had the skills you have now back then, you would have done things differently.

Identify your biggest regrets. When I work with clients on moving on from their past, it can be very overwhelming. This is because they see so many regrets. It's often helpful to categorize these things. Working on patterns of behavior is often more helpful than working on individual regrets. In other words, break down your undesirable behavior. Try to come up with a solution for that behavior instead of putting things in a general category. For example, I should have just eaten the half donut and allowed myself the splurge. This is better than letting it ruin and upset my entire day. Identifying that as the problem is more helpful than trying to categorize why I took the second donut.

Move on. At some point, you have to accept that the past has happened, and you've done everything in your power to amend past mistakes. It's now time to move on and accept those events as part of your story. They've all contributed to making you who you are. Being grateful for those experiences allows you to move on and truly forgive yourself.

Practice self-praise. Often, we only cut ourselves down for every little thing we do wrong. Yet, we don't praise ourselves for everything we do right. In any given day, you are faced with thousands of food decisions, and for the most part, you generally make good ones. It is rare that you pat yourself on the back for the 1,263 times you *did not* have a piece of candy or skipped the temptations of fried foods. Yet, the one time you cave and have a cookie, you slam yourself in *self-prison*. You throw the book at yourself until you hate yourself and everyone who crosses your path for the rest of the day. Practice self-praise. You are worth it.

Now that I have highlighted these strategies, it is time to put them into practice. For starters, focus on all the good things you have done. I realize this is an overwhelming task for some of you, so start out small. Pay close attention to your actions for one day. You will be surprised by how many good choices you make in comparison to poor ones. In asking one of my clients to complete this task, she was shocked to see how often she was cheating herself. Let me share her story.

> Erica was an overachiever. She typically finished first at most things she started. Generally, she did an outstanding job at anything she set her mind toward accomplishing. It was no different when she set a goal to lose weight for a wedding. Erica

knew she had to be the picture-perfect bride on the picture-perfect wedding day. She needed everything to be perfect. Erica made herself crazy each and every day by highlighting all the things that she did not execute with perfection. She could have a flawless day but would spend hours beating herself up for the smallest, most irrelevant things. Here is a log of her morning and afternoon broken into good versus poor choices:

5:00 Erica hit snooze and missed her morning workout.

5:45 Erica woke up and made breakfast for her fiancé. He loved cinnamon toast with butter. This is what he ate every day, and up until now, this is what Erica would eat. Now that Erica was trying to lose weight, she had to stick with oatmeal and fruit. She didn't have time to measure the oatmeal

6:30- She got in the car and picked up her friend who she carpools with. They stopped for coffee. Her friend ordered a hazelnut latte with extra whip and a scone. Erica didn't get anything, but did take a sip of the latte.

7:15 Erica clocked in at work. As usual, there were donuts and bagels in the front office along with bowls of candy. Erica resisted.

12:00 Lunchtime. Erica had made it all morning without grazing on any of the tempting foods in the office, although she did not have her midday snack. She was a bit disappointed in herself for this. She enjoyed her lunch and felt satisfied.

1:00 Erica had not drank any water yet, so she was stressing about that. She quickly drank a bottle and tried to keep up with it.

3:00 Erica took an afternoon walk during a break to get some steps in. She came back to her desk and ate her snack from the morning that she skipped.

5:00 She drove home with her friend. They stopped at the grocery store to get some items for dinner. Erica was a bit hungry and ended up eating a few of the samples that the store was featuring. She felt very guilty, as she knew the calories were a waste, but she couldn't undo her poor decision.

6:00 Erica came home and made dinner. Everything was prepped and she stayed on task.

Good Choices, Poor Choices

As you can see, Erica is doing an outstanding job following the program. It takes a tremendous amount of willpower and determination to get through the day and stay on course. I would have lost it at the cinnamon toast. I mean, who can resist taking one bite of that with the butter all melted and the crust crispy and flaky? Erica didn't even think about how amazing of a task that was. She also didn't spend any time commending herself for the dozens of other things she had done right that day.

Instead, much like most people, Erica was feeling guilty for oversleeping and missing her morning workout. She spent the day torturing herself and questioning the caloric value of her morning oats. She was pissed at herself for not drinking more water. Over and over in her head, like a crime scene. How could someone be so disturbed over missing a workout when she did so many other things right? These irrelevant things that she did wrong weren't affecting her progress directly. The negativity she instilled in herself was affecting her attitude. This would eventually affect her progress.

By practicing self-praise, individuals can create a positive environment for themselves. This attitude could, in turn, affect their weight loss. Being positive and forgiving yourself for making mistakes is essential. We can become our worst enemies, so be sure to kiss and make up and always give yourself praise. There is plenty of hate in this world. Lucky for you, I am going to tell you how to protect yourself later, after we talk dinner.

11

Here's an Idea: Make Your Own Dinner

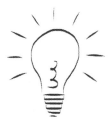

I'm guessing at this point you must be pretty hungry. We have talked about breakfasts, lunches, and snacks but not dinner. I wanted to give your brain a break before going into the very complicated dinner hour. Since you are still in kindergarten, we have to keep things simple. I am not going to get into the complicated cooking and meal-prepping techniques. That will be covered later once you graduate to second or third grade.

As difficult as it is for me to write this chapter without being offensive, some of the things I have to say may strike a nerve with some of you. If you are feeling pangs of electricity striking through your eyeballs and into your brain, then I am basically talking to you. If you are feeling nervous right now, then relaxxxxxxx … I am definitely talking to you, so just be a big kid and deal with it.

We live in a society where things are made so easy for us. My beloved grandmother lived to be ninety-seven. I was fortunate to have her in my life up until last year. She raised five children. Keep in mind, only a few turned out normal, but I'll leave my family drama out of this book and save it for my next novel *The Big, Fat Greek Family Fiasco*. (I left a few F-words out here to be nice.) Anyhow, my grandma had to actually bake the bread that she kneaded by hand. She let rise while she picked the green beans from the garden that she tended all summer long. I'm not kidding. What the fuck are we all bitching about?

My grandparents had to raise the flippin' chickens and wait for them to lay the Goddamn eggs for their kids to have breakfast. They would slaughter a chicken so they could serve it for dinner. I saw it happen, folks, and I never once heard my grandma complain about not having time to make dinner. To take it a step further, back in the 1950s, there were no convenience foods or frozen goods. If there were, most people didn't buy them. Our grandparents had to actually boil water to make the potatoes and couldn't just pop them in the microwave. We can take a meal that is basically complete and heat it up in three minutes, yet we don't have time to make dinner.

I'm not saying that I am completely off the hook on this one, but I have gotten better over the years. What made me realize how ridiculous I was by saying I didn't have time to make dinner was listening to all my clients bitch and whine about it. It is not a matter of not having time. It is a matter of not having the desire. Once I figured this out, it unlocked an entire world of knowledge to me about why people make excuses.

Why is it that people have such a hard time preparing dinner? Everyone claims they don't have time, whether they work during the day or not. There is never enough time to prepare dinner. I've had stay-at-home moms cry on my shoulder repeatedly, making claims that they just cannot get dinner made. I have also had people who work from home claim that there is absolutely no time to prep a meal for dinner. I'm sorry? I always wondered how I was able to cook for my family of six all while I worked full time. I ran a business, trained for marathons, and listened to this cockamamie bullshit all day long. This is where being me isn't always easy.

On the outside I have to kindly say: "Okay, Sondra, I know you are feeling overwhelmed with your daughter's cheer schedule, but let's plan how you can make a list to get things done."

But on the inside I am saying: "Are you fucking kidding me? How about you wake up at seven o'clock instead of nine o'clock and put some of the recipes I wrote for you in the fucking crockpot and turn it on before you leave all day to go shopping and bitch about how you have no time for jack shit."

Sorry, I knew that would happen. I may have a slight intolerance for people with poor time-management skills.

If you are being jolted right now, please take extra good notes during this chapter. Sondra really didn't want to make dinner. If she had any desire to have dinner on that table, she would have it done. The alternative to not having time to prepare a meal for her family was to order out or go out to eat.

Simple science: Sondra doesn't have time to make dinner, so she makes no effort to shop for ingredients or prepare for a meal. She hasn't even considered what options she has for dinner choices. She's basically set herself up for failure. She has created this drama around it all to make herself feel better about being a lazy ass. Sondra ended up being kind of crazy. Like the bat-shit-crazy kind of crazy that makes me love my job so much. I can only hope that she's reading this book right now wondering if I am talking about her and her fucked-up crazy ass. I guess no one will know but me. #Sondrawascrazy

The drama people create around how busy they are is usually a crock of shit. Unless you work for NASA or you are the president of the United States, I am pretty sure you can put the fucking chicken in the oven and feed your family. It's not that hard, people … Take the chicken that is already plucked for you and put it in the Goddamn oven. That's it. Since I get too angry when I talk about Sondra, I am going to share one of my favorite moments. When I coach people in learning how to prep meals, I often share this story.

Here is another story of a lady who couldn't seem to figure out how to get dinner on the table.

Carissa worked from home. She had two children and a very supportive husband who also enjoyed eating healthy. Despite all her efforts, Carissa would inevitably end up ordering out or going out for dinner. This occurred five out of the seven nights each week. This contributed to her inability to lose weight, as it was impossible for her to stay on her food plan. The restaurant menu choices were too tempting.

Carissa had a very hectic schedule and was on conference and sales calls all day. She had no time to cook, so she ordered out all the time. One day, Carissa was complaining to her amazing, super-cool, Greek goddess of a trainer. Carissa was upset because she just didn't have time to prepare dinner. Her trainer explained to her that she should put a few chicken breasts in the oven and let them cook. She reminded Carissa that this process would only take a few minutes. She could add a simple veggie to the chicken have a home-cooked meal. Carissa thought that was a great idea and was willing to give it a try.

The next week when Carissa came to her session, her trainer asked her how it went with eating. Carissa admitted to me—I mean, she told her trainer—that she didn't do well. She couldn't manage her time to make meals. One day her trainer—okay, it was me. I gave her another idea and suggested that the day she bought the chicken, she should come home and put several breasts in the oven, making them in advance for the week. This way, she would have the base for salads, sandwiches, wraps, and even dinner.

"Put the chicken in the oven, Carissa. Put the frickin' chicken in the oven!" I stood there in my ugly navy-blue training uniform and scolded her. "For the love of God, Carissa. Just open the flippin' oven door and throw the goddamn chicken in."

Week after week, Carissa came with some excuse for why she couldn't put the damn chicken in the oven.

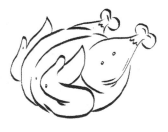

At this point, I just could not figure out why Carissa couldn't do this. One day the light bulb went on, and I figured it out. Carissa *did not want to put the frickin' chicken in the oven.* She didn't *want* to cook it because that would mean she would have to eat healthier and not eat out all the time. Because she didn't want to give up her restaurant habits, she convinced herself she had no time.

You see, Carissa had the time to put the chicken in the oven, but she told herself that she didn't. People don't like change, and Carissa wasn't ready to give up her restaurant visits. She told herself she didn't have time. I had to point this out to her. Putting chicken in the oven takes zero time. You open the door, put the chicken in, and walk away. Once Carissa realized this, and she decided she was ready to make this change she successfully put the chicken in the oven.

The message is clear in this story. Carissa clearly had time to take the chicken out of the package and place it in the oven. She could turn the oven on by pushing a button. She then had to walk away and do absolutely nothing for about forty-five minutes until it was done. Her fancy oven probably even beeped or shuts off when the chicken was done so Carissa didn't have to do jack shit. This was apparently still too much work not just for Carissa but for anyone who has ever bitched about not having time to make dinner. Carissa, along with thousands of others, would much rather pack her kids up on a cold night after a long day and drive to a crowded restaurant. They would rather wait an hour or longer for a sodium-filled, over-priced meal—a meal that is loaded with an astronomical number of calories that they don't need. They would rather do this than just put the flippin' chicken in the oven.

We're talking hours wasted every single day waiting for food to be served. Served to people who swear they don't have time to cook. It is such an astonishing thought process. Yet, it is one that most of us have convinced ourselves is legitimate. It almost makes me wish I could bring everyone back to the early 1900s just for one day, so we can have a full appreciation of how easy we have it. Next time you are at the grocery store, pay extra close attention to how easy it truly is. You are not climbing any trees to pick the apples for your kids' lunches. You aren't milking the cows for your fancy smoothies. You also are not hunting down the cows to put the beef on the table. Get over yourself, throw the shit in the Instant Pot, and push the Goddamn button. Dinner is served.

We have now established that you actually do have time to make dinner. Why is it that you are avoiding this not-so-difficult task? I'll rephrase that question. What causes people to avoid completing tasks that they dislike? What reasons do you have for not having dinner prepared? Your answers are probably very similar to those from the people I surveyed. An online study revealed some interesting information. One hundred participants were asked why they don't have dinner ready for their families. These were the top results in order of popularity.

Reason 1: "I don't have time." We just went over this. There may certainly be true circumstances in which someone does not have time to prepare a gourmet meal. However, there are always a few simple *dinner tricks* that you can pull out of your magic bag in these situations. These can be used on nights that you have bullshitted yourself and everyone else into believing that you didn't have time to cook. The beautiful part of this is that no one has to know. You can continue to blah, blah, blah about how fucking busy you are all you fucking want. As long as you get food on the table, no one will care. Don't go getting too excited just yet. These dinner tricks require a bit of work and prep, so you can't be a total lazy ass. My God ...

Dinner Tricks for those Who
(Think They) Lack Time

1. When you do finally get around to making a meal (which I will help you with, of course), you can always make two. It does not take any extra time to buy double the ingredients and make double the recipe. This works great with casseroles or anything that you can freeze. Most meals can be made in advance and frozen. Crockpot meals can be stored in Ziplock bags uncooked and thrown in the crockpot that morning. I always make double batches of enchilada casseroles, lasagna dishes, and veggie casseroles. If you know you have one of these meals ready to go in the freezer for those busy days, it can be a lifesaver!

2. Breakfast for dinner. Why not? One of the easiest and fastest things that you can whip up is an omelet. You just have to make sure you always have eggs on hand. You don't have to be fancy. If you have some of your favorite veggies on hand, even if frozen, you can put together a hearty omelet in less than ten minutes. If you're prepared and you have cheese on hand, this very satisfying meal will fill you up and keep you trim.

3. Always have your protein cooked and ready. If you put your chicken in the oven and cook up a large quantity of it, the work is done for the week. You now don't have to work as hard to thaw out the chicken, season it, and cook it. It's done. Most recipes can be prepared in minutes if the chicken is already cooked. I like to always keep fixings for a Mexican dish in the pantry—canned corn, black beans, refried beans, salsa, and tortillas. If the chicken is cooked, you could easily make tacos or a casserole. An enchilada bake or a variety of different things with the ingredients that you already have can also be whipped up in no time.

Reason 2: "I don't have the things I need to cook." Well there's only one way to fix that … Get your kitchen ready and equipped for meal making. Sorry, but I'm not sorry that people haven't figured out that you can go to the damn store and buy things to use to help you cook. Isn't that crazy? Who knew? You can buy these things to make cooking possible so you don't have to go out to eat every single night?! So, what things are needed? I am guessing if you are reading this book, you don't live in a tent and have an oven with pots and pans, so no lesson needed there … Can openers and spatulas? Nope, you have those too … So what *things* are needed? This will vary from person to person. It will depend on what foods you and your family like. The items should be foods that can be stored for a long time either on the shelf or in the freezer. This is not an impossible task to accomplish. Be sure to keep preservatives low and nutritional quality high. These staple items should always be on hand so that you can whip a meal together even in a pinch. Always be sure you watch the sodium levels of some of these items and select the lowest option available. Here is a list of some of my suggested staple ingredients. All these items can be purchased in bulk, they can kept on hand, and they are very versatile for cooking.

Spices and Condiments

- garlic powder
- oregano
- minced garlic
- olive oil
- spray oil
- onion powder
- chili powder

Canned Goods

+ tuna

+ chicken

+ corn

+ black beans

+ garbanzo beans

+ kidney beans

+ refried beans

+ tomato paste

+ crushed tomatoes

Jarred Goods

+ salsa

+ olives

+ pickles

+ tomato sauce

+ light salad dressings

+ marinades

+ barbeque sauces

Frozen Foods

+ chicken

- beef
- fish
- assorted vegetables
- cubed potatoes

Other

- bags of dry beans
- rice
- quinoa
- pasta

Reason 3: "I don't know what to make." Part of me feels sorry for people who say this, and the other part of me wants to kick them in the throat. Come on … If you were born yesterday, then maybe I would buy this excuse. If you just arrived to planet Earth from fucking Jupiter, and you have no clue what a Goddamn recipe is, then I will grant you forgiveness. If you just fell out of the sky because Jack and his giant beanstalk have kept you hostage for the last three decades, you get a pass. But you were not a beanstalk-farming slave. It's time to put this book down and seek professional help.

I guess what I am trying to say is that there are no reasons at all for why someone should not know what to prepare for dinner. If you live alone and you are unsure of what to make, then I will ask you to join the beanstalk farmers, as they just exited the room. If you have a family and don't know what to make, then maybe you should ask them. It's not that hard. The next time you talk to them, just mention food and ask them to tell you what they would like to eat. I am guessing you have probably seen them eat this type of food before; after all, you do live with them.

Once you have this figured out, you can find all these crazy amazing ways to cook dinner on this magical new place called the interweb. You know, Facechat, Instabook, Snapagram, Pinterchat, Tinderweb, and Web PhD can get you any information you need. Be resourceful. Pretend there is a flash sale at Ulta or Nordstrom, get your ass online, and figure out how to make dinner. There are *millions* of recipes available online. You can even narrow down your searches by putting in keywords such as "quick easy healthy dinners" or "idiot-proof dinner recipes." Nonetheless, get your head out of your ass and get it on the internet instead. Save a bunch of easy recipes and have them ready for those dinner emergencies as needed.

Reason 4: "Everyone in my family eats different things." I'm mother of four who has always worked full time. My sexy, hot husband may be awesome, but he's picky as shit. I can only say that if you are someone who uses this as an excuse, then it's your own damn fault. Once again, I must apologize for my bold and forward tone, but I never said I would sugarcoat things in this book.

I have four kids—four fucking monsters. I love, them of course, but motherhood wouldn't be as fun if you couldn't publish a book and call your children monsters. It's not so bad now. At its worst, my husband wouldn't eat anything green that crunched. Then he lovingly asked me to follow his 40/30/30 macro plan when making dinner. Meanwhile, our thirteen-year-old would eat anything you would put in front of her as long as it was in the form of soup. My eleven-year-old decided she wanted to be vegan. My nine-year-old boy only ate carbs, and the two-year-old inherited my celiac disease and can't have anything with wheat. It was always fun for me to come home from work and figure this out after listening to people bitch all day long about how they just couldn't handle dinnertime. I always figured it out. Guess what else? It wasn't even hard. Guess what else, else? I am going to tell you all about it so you can no longer use this as an excuse.

If you are a beanstalk farmer, you should probably come back and pay attention to the rest of this chapter. If you are still wondering if you are too much like Sondra, don't worry about that for now ...

Cooking for One, Cooking for All

No matter how complex your family's needs are, you can have a dinner plan. For example, maybe you will make a Mexican dish. You can provide a variety of fixings that all family members can enjoy. Since you are watching your calories, then you can skip the cheese and sour cream. If your daughter is vegetarian, then she can make her dish with just the beans and no meat. If your son won't eat vegetables, then he can have his with the chicken and cheese. You can do this with a variety of meals. Provide the protein, a vegetable, and a carb, and allow members of your family to construct their meals accordingly.

Don't create monsters. There is a certain extent of entitlement here on the part of your family. If you have always catered to their needs, they will naturally expect you to provide all these special accommodations for them. When my brother and I grew up, we were stuck eating some of the most ethnic Greek dishes that used to make my spine chill. We're talking octopus and squid, lamb and smelt dishes, and salmon meals where we had to pick the bones out of every bite. I don't really remember thinking, "Awesome, Mom! We're having feta and lamb liver sausage for dinner tonight!" But we ate it. I do not recall a single dish that wasn't consumed, as strange and un-American as they all were. We were not given the choice that many of us give our kids today, which is only doing them an injustice. Looking back at those feta lamb sausages and octopus meals, I should be so lucky to have my mom cooking like that for me every day ... and she totally would! #ihavethebestmom #iloveoctopus

Involve your family. Put the ball in their court. Have the family help make food-planning decisions for the week. If you communicate which dinners work best for your family, then you can plan for those meals. Having the family involved will include them in the process. This will help them realize how much work is involved in this process. This understanding will give them a level of respect for the time and effort that is taken every single day. This is also a great way to role model this positive behavior to your children. Understanding the importance of meal planning and healthy living is a great thing to teach your children.

As a little kindergartener, I feel compelled to give you a basic dinner outline. You should follow this while constructing your evening meals. Looking back to chapter 6 when we learned about the must-haves, let me review them and revise them for dinner options.

Must-Haves

Protein

20–25 grams will help sustain your hunger until you can eat again.

+ chicken
+ lean beef
+ fish
+ lean pork
+ beans
+ cottage cheese
+ eggs

Complex Carbohydrates

30–40 grams of complex carbs.

- quinoa
- whole-grain rice
- sweet potato
- potato
- pasta
- polenta
- grains

Healthy Fat

8–10 grams of a healthy fat.

- avocado
- avocado oil
- olives
- olive oil
- grape seed oil
- egg yolk
- coconut
- coconut oil
- nuts
- nut butter

Just like for the breakfast meals, it is important that you include each category in all your dinners. Constructing a meal with 4–6 ounces of protein, 30 grams of carbohydrates, and 10 grams of fat is ideal. You should include vegetables in your meal to add substance and flavor. This is an advanced-level move and not on the kindergarten curriculum. Most vegetables fall into the category of a carbohydrate. Always know that you can include unlimited green or white vegetables, as they are generally low in calories. I will include some of my favorite recipes in the appendix of this very awesome book for you to enjoy. Before you get too excited, I have to teach you how to compose your dinner plate. After all, a kindergartener could never do this by themselves. She would most likely not only make a mess but also pile too much crap on her plate.

Designing the Perfect Dinner Plate

This is what it all boils down to. Figuring out what to put on your plate and walking away from the crockpot. You almost have to pretend that you are at a restaurant and that you get what you get. Nothing more. This is the part of the dinnertime ritual that will need the most willpower and diligence. Often, I suggest to my clients that they should plan what they are going to put on their plates before they start spooning stuff on. Have a rough idea of what you are going to eat, the portions, and even the caloric values of each one. Properly nourish your body and have a high-protein snack going into this dangerous part of the day. You are less likely to bulldoze food on your plate as if it is your last meal. Never ever invite the gargoyles to supper. They will jump off your shoulder and onto your dinner plate. They will chant and sing at the top of their lungs every time they see you losing control. It's like a fucking gargoyle Super Bowl party. It doesn't matter who is stuffing her face … All the gargoyles come out to cheer.

Once you have a plan, you need to try and stick to it. If you are logging, have the meal logged already. You are less likely to deviate from the plan once you have it entered in. Less likely. Now it is time to put the food on your plate. Here is where people fail. The reason why you overeat and gain weight at dinnertime may have nothing to do with the type of foods that you are eating. Your home-cooked meal may be perfectly nutritious. The culprit here may be a totally invisible factor that is causing you to overeat.

Your portion sizes may be too big, and the way you arrange your plate may be the reason why. As basic as it sounds, setting the arrangement of your plate will change the way you compose your food.

I discovered this completely on accident one Thanksgiving when I was putting plates together for myself and my daughter. When I made my plate, I went for the salad first. I piled on the greens. Later, I added some of my mom's delicious olive-oil-marinated green beans, some baked zucchini, then some turkey, and finally some mashed potatoes. Perfecto. When I made my daughter's plate, I filled it as she requested: mashed potatoes, Greek Pastichio (a pasta casserole), sweet potatoes, turkey, green beans, and salad. It didn't even phase me initially, but as I was trying to fit salad on her plate, there wasn't a whole lot of room left. I figured she could always go up for seconds.

As I sat down and ate my meal, I noticed that I dove into the salad first. So good. My palate had been covered in the flavors of the delicious, crisp vegetables and fresh ingredients. So, so good. I was enjoying the salad so much that it took a while to hit up the other foods. When I did take a bite of my mom's heaven-in-a-spoonful mashed potatoes, they were amazing. Interestingly, I really wanted more salad. This was perfect. I had just the right balance of carbohydrates and proteins on my plate, along with an abundance of vegetables to keep me munching. I looked around at everyone else's overflowing plates. I realized that had I loaded mine up with those delicious sweet potatoes before I left room for the leans and greens, I would have undoubtedly eaten them first. This would instantly make me a *dinner overeater*, which is a condition that cannot be reversed once you have been diagnosed.

dinner

noun often attributive

din·ner | \ˈdi-nər \

Definition of dinner

    1a: the principal meal of the day. having dinner at five o'clock

    b: a formal feast or banquet held a dinner in her honor

    2: TABLE D'HÔTE sense 2

    3: the food prepared for a dinner eat your dinner

overeat

verb

over·eat | \ ˌō-vər-ˈēt \

overate\ ˌō-vər-'āt \; overeaten\ ˌō-vər-'ē-t³n \;overeating

Definition of overeat

intransitive verb

: to eat to excess

Synonyms

gorge, gormandize, pig out, swill

Based on these definitions taken from the *Merriam-Webster Dictionary*, if you are a dinner overeater, this basically means you eat too much. Some signs to look for if you feel you may suffer from this condition include:

+ You feel pretty full, but you are still eating and not planning on stopping anytime soon.

+ You no longer taste the food. In fact, you don't even enjoy the flavor anymore.

+ You need to take a break because you are physically tired from chewing and shoveling food into your mouth.

+ You get a midmeal hot flash. This is not a good sign.

+ Your pants suddenly don't fit. You find yourself wishing you would have worn your baggiest pants and now have lost circulation from the waist down.

- ✦ You think you will actually die if you do not remove yourself from the table and lie down immediately.

- ✦ You go back for seconds and are already planning your game plan for your third trip.

- ✦ You try to justify the enormous amounts of foods that you are inhaling to the other dinner guests. You say things like, "I barely ate today," and, "I have been so good. I have been waiting for this all week."

- ✦ You find yourself covering your extended belly with a coach pillow when you sit down after dinner.

Some physical symptoms you may feel are:

- ✦ restlessness

- ✦ excitability

- ✦ irritability

- ✦ agitation

- ✦ dizziness

- ✦ headache

- ✦ fear

- ✦ anxiety

- ✦ agitation

- ✦ tremor

- weakness

- blurred vision

- sleep problems (insomnia)

- dry mouth or unpleasant taste in the mouth

- diarrhea

- constipation

- stomach pain

- nausea

- vomiting

- fever

- hair loss

- loss of appetite

- weight loss

- loss of interest in sex

- impotence

- difficulty having an orgasm

- increase blood pressure

- increased heart rate

- heart palpitations

I am trying to be funny. These are actual side effects of a prescription amphetamine used to treat attention deficit disorder. My guess is by looking at that awful list, probably 80 percent of it rings true to overeating. Having this condition at any point during the day is an undesirable and uncomfortable situation. Putting yourself in this position during the dinner hour is especially dangerous. You are filling your stomach up with a large quantity of food and then going straight to bed where you are not moving for seven to eight hours. You are also lying down, which can cause complications with digestion and breathing. People who suffer from acid reflux or IBS need to have this food digest before having it sit in a sedentary state for several hours. No matter how you look at it, it is not good.

The purpose of each meal is to provide enough nourishment to get you to the next meal. You are not a bear. It is not winter. You are not hibernating. Eat for energy. Don't eat solely for pleasure. You will eventually be able to find the right balance and be able to synthesize the two. Pretend your dinner has been prepared by a world-famous chef. Cherish every bite and enjoy the flavor. Do not inhale it, and you will find a whole new experience in flavors of food. Enjoy the textures and the temperatures.

12

Beat the Bloat:
Sodium and Water

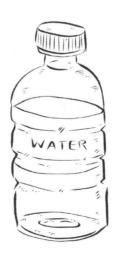

Are you overwhelmed yet? You should be. The shit is overwhelming. If it were easy, everyone would look like Jennifer Aniston, and there would be no multimillion-dollar industry. There would be no need for a chapter 12 in this book, and you and I would both be able to do something else right now. Instead, I have to educate you on hydration, and you have to keep reading about just another thing that needs to be modified in your life.

Don't be so sad … Water is amazing. Water is refreshing and revitalizing. Once you start drinking it regularly, you will crave it. You will see the benefits of hydration from your skin to your nails to your mind clarity, and you will never want to give it up.

I always wondered why it is so important to drink water when you are trying to lose weight. It makes zero sense. They say you should drink water, and that will speed up your metabolism. They say water will flush your system and help you burn calories. They say if you drink water, you will lose weight faster. First of all, who the fuck is *they*? Secondly, how does all of this work?

Let me explain.

Drinking water helps boost your metabolism, cleanses your body of waste, and acts as an appetite suppressant. Also, drinking more water helps your body stop retaining water, leading you to drop those extra pounds of water weight. Here's what you can do to help encourage weight loss:

Drink water before you eat. Because water is an appetite suppressant, drinking it before meals can make you feel fuller, therefore reducing the amount of food you eat. Drinking water before just one meal per day would cause you to ingest 27,000 fewer calories per year. Do the math: you'd lose about eight pounds per year just from drinking water. Now imagine if you drank it before each meal.

Replace calorie-filled drinks with water. Ditch the sodas and juice and replace them with water to help you lose weight. If you think water tastes boring, add a slice of lemon. A glass of water with lemon is a recipe for successful weight loss because the pectin in lemons helps reduce food cravings. If you think water doesn't really help with weight loss, give up those sugary drinks for just a few weeks and see the difference.

Drink it ice-cold. Drinking ice-cold water helps boost your metabolism because your body has to work harder to warm the water up, therefore burning more calories and helping you to lose weight. Plus, ice-cold water is just so much more refreshing than water that's room temperature.

Drink enough water. If you really want the water you drink to help you lose weight, you should follow the 8 x 8 rule recommended by most nutritionists: Drink eight, 8-ounce glasses of water per day for weight loss and to maintain an ideal weight. You might need to drink more water if you exercise a lot or sweat heavily or less water if you drink other beverages like herbal tea (make sure they are decaffeinated). How do you know if you're getting enough water? A general rule is to check the toilet after you've gone to the bathroom. You'll know you're well hydrated if your urine is clear or very light yellow in color. The darker your urine, the more water you need to drink, especially if weight loss is your goal.

Being dehydrated can mess with your mental, physical, and emotional health. Numerous studies show attention, memory, and mood can be damaged, and physical distress such as headaches, constipation, and kidney problems can result. It's not hard. Just drink the damn water. I have found that people who dislike water end up craving it after they build it into their routines.

Water is also the best way to combat bloat—you know, bloat. That fantabulous condition that occurs after you have consumed a meal that is high in sodium and may cause water retention. Fucking bloat. You could be having the best week.

One bad decision later, and you are looking at a potbelly the size of fricking watermelon and hands the size of baseball mitts. One would think that if you are retaining water that you should stop drinking water until you've lost the fluids your body is holding on to. Wrong answer.

Since our bodies like to fuck with us and make us crazy, this would be far too easy of a solution. Instead, it is just the opposite. In order for the body to release the fluid it is retaining, you have to give it more fluid to get it to release all of the water that it is retaining. I have this mental image of Niagara Falls in my head. The water just builds up until it has to spill over and finally flush out. If you have ever experienced edema (fancy name for bloat), once your body decides to release the water, you are in the bathroom every hour. You become a peeing machine. It's the best. The puffiness goes away with each trip to the toilet—your face, your hands, and your feet. I have felt like I had one of those sumo wrestler Halloween costume suits on at eight o'clock in the morning, and by noon I've been back to my normal self. Water!

You may be wondering what causes this bloat. This is a complex question, but I will keep it at a kindergarten level. Most likely, the culprit is sodium. That's right, people. If things weren't already hard enough, now you have to watch sodium. Sad but true. You have to add this to this mix, but it really is the least of your worries. If you can manage all the shit I already threw at you, counting sodium milligrams is nothing.

Why does eating foods high in salt make you bloated? Sodium imbalances potassium. Sodium is well absorbed by cells and brings water in with it. Thus, when you eat a large amount of sodium, it can cause cells to temporarily retain water until balance can be restored to cellular fluid levels. This is also why when you restrict sodium intake, water retention decreases. That's the sixth-grade explanation. The kindergarten version is much more basic. Table salt is the most common cause of water retention. Excess sodium makes the body hold extra fluids in the cells. When you cut down salt and high-sodium condiments, you can quickly lose water weight.

I have had clients see an eight-pound water fluctuation from consuming a high-sodium meal. Although this does not mean they have gained eight pounds of fat, their bodies have indeed gained eight pounds of fluid. The bad news is that you can probably see this weight, as it is retained and is visible. The good news is that it can be lost as quickly as in one day by drinking water and flushing it out. Most people would take a few days to drop eight pounds of water weight, but that number is unusual. Typically, someone who eats offtrack may see a three-pound weight gain. This could drop relatively fast. I have clients who have become completely derailed by this water gain. Instead of getting back on track and losing the water weight, they go right into self-sabotage mode and let the wrecking ball start destructing.

Most foods that are not on your program might be higher in sodium than what you are used to eating. If you eat out, you might as well suck on a salt cube. Even the healthiest options at the healthiest restaurants have sodium levels well over 2,000 milligrams for one entrée. Why is this? Unless you are at a farm-to-table restaurant, most places preserve their ingredients, causing the sodium levels to skyrocket.

Once my husband and I went out just for appetizers since we were being calorie conscious. I looked up the menu at a well-known restaurant and planned my entire day around this treat. I had just lost my baby weight from baby number four and finally squeezed my ass into these black True Religion jeans that I paid way too much for. No dinner, just appetizers. We had a sitter just for a short time, and we were going to go home and have a home-cooked healthy meal. Our waitress came and brought us the bread that we didn't eat. We ordered drinks—wine for me and a beer for him. The steamed mussels and crab legs with no butter were the lowest in calories on the menu. Lord knows I spent all week researching which restaurant in town would have appetizers that would fit the criteria needed for my strict True Religion standards. The appetizers arrived. Delicious. I sat there and watched all the tables around me getting served. I savored the small bites of my mini meal as I witnessed thousands of calories being devoured at the tables around me. I felt empowered that I was having an enjoyable evening with my hot husband eating my delicious treat and knowing that it wasn't derailing me.

As the hour went on, I noticed my rings started to feel tight. I figured it must have been the temperature of the restaurant and continued to eat my butterless crabmeat. Suddenly, I felt thirsty as well and patiently waited for our waitress to fill my water. My hot husband and I finished our appetizers, paid the bill, drank more water, and headed home. A victory! We went out—a night out without our monsters, and we stayed on track with our eating.

The next morning, I woke up and felt like I had sandpaper in my mouth. Don't laugh. I could have filed my nails with my tongue and sanded off my calluses with the roof of my mouth. My hands felt tight, and my face looked puffy. Dumbfounded, it didn't bother me because I knew I stayed on track the day before. I got up, used the bathroom, and brushed my teeth. Next on the list was the daily weigh-in. Excited to hop on the scale after a good eating day, I skipped on with confidence and grace. If there were a camera in the bathroom to capture my reaction, I would have definitely included the image of my face on this page. To best describe it, it was somewhere between Macaulay Culkin putting aftershave on his face in *Home Alone* and Michael Douglas finding his pet rabbit cooking on his stove in *Fatal Attraction*. I had gained four pounds! Four frickin pounds. I should have known when I took my jeans off and I had imprints of the stitching down my leg. The Goddamn True Religion logo was sketched in my ass until the next morning, all $175 of it.

I quickly jumped off the scale.

I looked right at myself in the mirror and said some choice things and then ran upstairs.

I logged on to the interweb to look up the nutritional information of the foods that had poisoned me.

The calories were spot on.

The sodium, not so much.

How didn't I notice this?

The steamed mussels contained 2,116 milligrams for each serving. The appetizer had four servings. The crab legs were 3,792 milligrams for the one pound that we shared. The pound was only 387 calories. That was what I looked at. Little did I know that I had consumed close to 8,000 milligrams of sodium, which is close to four days' worth. No wonder I looked like the fucking Michelin Man with a high-end jean logo imprinted on my ass.

If I didn't know better, I would have gone straight to the pancake mix and started mixing.

That's right, kids. Mama is making pancakes for breakfast, and she is going to eat all the scraps that you monsters leave behind. Where is that damn wrecking ball?

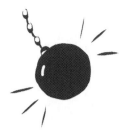

However, I knew better. I knew it was water. I knew it was not fat. I knew that if I drank water and stayed on my plan, my body would drop that retention, and I would be myself again. I also knew I would never eat mussels and crab legs ever again, not even if I was about to starve to death. F that.

After a few days, my weight came back down, and I avoided self- sabotage. I learned from my mistake and now always check the sodium content of all foods. It has been fascinating to learn how many healthy foods are very high in sodium. Americans eat on average about 3,400 milligrams of sodium per day. However, the Dietary Guidelines for Americans recommends limiting sodium intake to less than 2,300 milligrams per day. That is equal to about 1 teaspoon of salt. Individuals with blood pressure issues should get far less than that, so watching sodium intake is essential.

Here are some of the foods that are highest in sodium levels and that should be avoided or eaten in moderation. Some of these foods mat surprise you!

Foods High in Sodium

+ yeast breads

+ pizza

+ all lunchmeat sandwiches

+ cold cuts and cured meats

+ burritos and tacos

+ soups, unless homemade

+ all savory snacks

+ chicken, rotisserie

+ cheeses

+ cottage cheese

+ pasta mixed dishes

+ mixed seasonings

+ bacon, frankfurters, and sausages

+ other Mexican mixed dishes

+ tomato-based condiments

+ salad dressings

+ poultry mixed dishes

+ all soda and soft drinks

+ all ready-to-eat cereal

+ mashed potatoes and white potato mixtures

+ fish and seafood

+ french fries

+ Chinese food

+ soy sauce

+ pickles and olives

While this list is useful to know, it doesn't mean you must avoid all of these foods. Instead, follow these five tips to help you select the foods with the least amount of sodium. Remember, starting small can make a big difference. Always look foods up before you eat them, and drink your water.

13

Be True to You: Mindless Eating and Logging

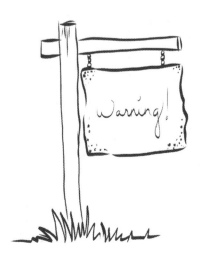

Always look up foods before you eat!

Always. Don't fool yourself, and don't be a fool.

I think about back when people didn't know what calories were. How great was the world back then? People just ate and didn't think about the caloric value of foods. Back then people were not overweight. They used food for fuel, and eventually, they figured out that food gave them energy. They ate when they needed energy.

We eat when we need energy too. We also eat when we are bored, when we are thirsty, and when we are stressed. We have learned to eat for entertainment. We are taught to eat at social gatherings. We feel the need to stuff our faces at every event whether we are hungry or not. Our bodies don't burn all of the fuel that is provided from this food. This fuel then turns to fat. This fat now sits on your ass, and it causes you to stress eat. Now you are trapped in this terrible cycle. You are trapped with your fat and your food and your stress. Round and round you go, eating and stressing, adding more and more fat to your already fat ass.

"I have fallen, and I can't get up!"

Get up!

It is time.

It is time to be true to yourself.

In order to do this, you need to start seeing things as they truly are. A large majority of people do not realize why they are overweight. This is because they are in denial about what they are actually eating. If you think you are not guilty of this, I call bullshit. After twenty years of logging my food, I still find myself underestimating the number of calories I shove down my throat.

Unless you look it up and write it down, you are wasting your time. I have seen this happen 23,876 times, and that was just last month. I am going to cover a few topics in this chapter. I cannot stress their importance. The rest of everything else you have learned will mean nothing if you fight me on what is next.

If you do anything I tell you to do, for the love of God, log your food, and do it accurately.

When I started my first food journal, I had to look shit up in a book. Like I mentioned earlier, I had this food encyclopedia that had the caloric values of foods listed in alphabetical order. This was in the eighties, so I am unsure how accurate these figures even were. To top it off, food manufacturers were not required to provide nutritional information on labels. It is a hard concept to imagine, but the sugar-coated cereal we ate as kids had zero proof of how damaging it was to our health. Those were the days …

Back then, we could blame other things for our weight gain. Today, it stares at us right in the face. Not only is everything labeled, but we have apps that tell us the exact calories of foods. Restaurants provide this information on their websites and even on their menus. Many of them have the caloric values of each entrée posted right beside each line item on the wall. You can see the damage before you even order. It is shocking that people will still order the fancy-dancy Frappuccino for 850 calories even though it's $7.50. Once again, the CEOs of these companies have to be laughing somewhere out on their yachts. I can just see them as they developed his insane idea: "Let's make an iced coffee that is really a milkshake and charge a shit ton of money for it to see who will buy it."

There's a multibillion-dollar idea that made my job harder.

People drink this coffee because it's good. They don't log it because it's coffee. Everyone knows that coffee has no calories. How bad could it be?

Let's ask Alyky who found out the hard way.

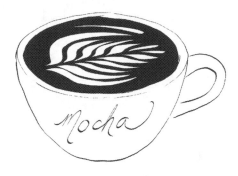

Alyky was a true coffee lover. She had been a coffee drinker as long as she could remember. Alyky could drink coffee any way it is served. Hot or cold. Cream or black. Fancy or plain. It didn't matter to Alyky. What mattered was that she started her day with a large cup. When Alyky got pregnant, she had to reduce the amount of coffee she drank due to the caffeine. She switched to decaf and made it through the nine months. As soon as her sweet baby girl was born, she went back to enjoying her morning cup of java. She had one large black cup each morning. Every afternoon she treated herself to a large mocha from the local coffee shop. This was her daily splurge to herself, and she never added sugar or whipped cream.

Alyky worked really hard to lose her baby weight. She worked out and watched everything she ate. She tried to record and log most things that she consumed. She knew she was doing a great job, as she had lost forty of the fifty-five pounds she had gained while pregnant. Months had gone by, yet she could not get the last fifteen pounds off. She was already exercising daily. She knew her eating was spot on. She could not figure it out. Alyky was reading an article one day about weight loss and the metabolism. She stumbled across some research that indicated how people who log what they eat are more likely to lose weight. Alyky was kind of logging but knew she was not logging everything she ate. She had not been logging little things like condiments or green vegetables. She also never logged her coffee. That is when it dawned on her.

She quickly ran to her computer to try and figure out how many calories were in her midday mocha indulgence. This was during a time before smartphones and WiFi, so she had to wait for the dinosaur dial-up to log on to the web. Thank goodness for AOL, she was able to do some quick research. A large mocha without the whipped cream had 580 calories. She quickly remembered all of the times that she forgot to skip the whip. On those occasions, she was blessed with a 620-calorie treat. She recalled the handful of times that she splurged and stopped for a second mocha. White mocha, peppermint mocha, Goddamn mocha was spread all over her thighs, and she had no idea. Although 580 calories isn't terrible, the problem was that it wasn't a meal. It lacked nutrition. It didn't have the proper component needed to nurture her body. It was a big waste of almost 600 calories every day, and she was pissed. Furthermore, it was one-third of her caloric allowance for the day, which she was mindlessly exceeding. Once Alyky became aware of everything she was doing, she dropped that last fifteen pounds. It really did melt off, like mocha.

That was twenty years ago. Alyky still loves her coffee. She stopped drinking mochas every day since it wasn't worth the calories or the money. Her baby is now a college student and works part time as a barista. She makes an amazing no-whip, sugar-free, low-fat, skinny mocha with almond milk for her mom. It's only 125 calories. It is a daily project for her to make heathier drinks for people when they come in, as more and more people are aware of the calories in some of these drinks today. #dailyprojects

Mindless. You see that is the key word. Mindless. We all do it. Often, we are mindless because we want to be. It is easier to look the other way and ignore the reality of what we are actually doing. The grown-up term for this is denial. When someone is in denial, she refuses to believe something is true. Being mindless is the act of doing something without giving it any thought.

denial

de·ni·al

/dəˈnīəl/

noun

the action of declaring something to be untrue.

"she shook her head in denial"

synonyms: contradiction, refutation, rebuttal, repudiation, disclaimer

the refusal of something requested or desired.

"the denial of insurance to people with certain medical conditions"

mind·less

/ˈmīn(d)ləs/

adjective

adjective: mindless

acting or done without justification or concern for the consequences.

"a generation of mindless vandals"

synonyms: stupid, idiotic, brainless, imbecilic, imbecile, asinine, witless, foolish, empty-headed

Mindless behavior and denial go hand in hand. If you are being mindless about what you are eating, most likely you are also denying this behavior. I would also bet that you are blaming your thyroid or hormones on your weight gain. Instead, you should get your head out of your ass and start logging everything you eat.

It is impossible to snap someone out of this state of denial. You can't logic with someone who doesn't see that she is at fault for something. In order to prove someone wrong, you have to prove her wrong. In this case, I suggest to my clients that they log every single thing they put in their mouths. No matter what.

This is the only way we can determine how many calories are consumed. Our minds play tricks on us. We block out the things that we don't want to remember. These things often include bites of cookies and nibbles of cheese. Hundreds of calories go undetected daily, as we mindlessly pick and graze on junk all day long. I played a mental game once. I wondered what my thighs would look like if I smeared all the crap I ate on them instead of mindlessly eating it throughout the day. A little cheese dip. Some sour cream. A few pieces of chocolate and some mini Oreos. The crust of frozen pizza and a few french fries. Some grapes and pretzels. The list continues. By the end of the day, my legs looked like an art deco mosaic nightmare. Actually, they looked like the bottom of a trash can. The calories totaled several hundred.

As soon as people begin diligently recording their food intake, they start seeing that they are overeating. This usually causes them to be more mindful of everything they put in their mouths. Next comes the result of weight loss. It is a foolproof solution. If you do not calculate the calories of the foods that you are eating, you are more likely to eat less when you record the food you eat. This simple task will make you more aware of what you are doing. Anyone who has ever eaten a sleeve of cookies can tell you. They would have stopped if they had to record every single cookie as they scoffed it down. Every person who has every lost weight has started with logging. The logging helps you avoid mindless eating. This will keep you from falling into a dangerous state of denial. It's like a Christmas miracle! Halleluiah!

Anytime you put yourself in a situation where you lose track of what you are eating, things become abstract. Abstract things are not able to be seen or measured. When things get to this point, you have most likely lost control. You no longer have any real way of measuring what you have eaten, and the damage is done. In other words, you're fucked.

Dining out is a luxury that is not only relaxing but very satisfying. It is one that many Americans have made a part of their weekly routines. Going to a restaurant with family or friends and having someone cook and serve food to you is a wonderful treat. This treat does not come without an expensive price tag. Obviously, you will have to pay for the food and service. You will also pay for the high-calorie extravaganza that comes with the pricey bill. The mindless eating and denial will accompany the delicious entrees and overpriced wine lists. From the time you sit down until the time you leave, your jaw is chomping. Unless you are on red alert and logging every bite, you will be in for a big surprise. My suggestion is to plan your restaurant outings. Look up the menu and even plan what you are going to eat before you get there. You may even choose to log what you plan on eating before you go. This will ensure that there will be no surprises.

My client Nikki had the surprise of her life after a night out with her husband. Although Nikki looked up the menu before she went, she did not log what she planned to eat beforehand. She learned from her mistake, and hopefully you will too.

Nikki didn't know that there were some unexpected guests joining them. Gargoyles love dining out. They super love getting dressed up and watching you make an ass of yourself in public. They especially love watching you pay extra for food that you have mindlessly eaten. By the way, if you are wondering, the gargoyles do dress up when they join you at restaurants. These assholes aren't from the ghetto; they like to travel high class.

Nikki was an energetic and athletic young lady who had just lost twenty-five pounds. She was training for her first marathon and had completed her very first ten-mile training run. She was incredibly proud of her accomplishment and was pleased with the progress of her training so far.

Her and her husband were celebrating their fifth wedding anniversary, so they made dinner plans after her run. Nikki spent most of her run thinking about what she was going to order and looking forward to the evening. She picked one of her favorite places to eat that night for two reasons. It was one of her favorites (I just said that), and they had a light menu. She did her homework and looked up all of her choices beforehand. She was good to go. She thought …

When she and her husband arrived at the restaurant, Nikki was feeling amazing. They went to the bar for a drink. She ordered a vodka with seltzer water and lime. A good choice. A woman at the bar noticed how fit Nikki was and commented on her muscular legs. Nikki always felt self-conscious about her frame, and this compliment was exactly what she needed to boost her self-esteem. Tonight was going to be a good night. She had run ten miles like a gazelle, she was down twenty-five pounds, and she was out enjoying her anniversary with her love. She could hear the beat from the song from the seventies band Queen "We Are the Champions" playing in her head as she sipped the 100-calorie beverage.

Vodka water … 105 calories (Imagine a little gargoyle dressed up in a tuxedo sitting on Nikki's shoulder entering numbers on his calculator right now.)

It was time to be seated. The bread came to the table. Pretzel loaf. Mothertrucker. She had looked this up. The calories were astronomical, so she treated herself to just a sliver. Since her husband was being romantic and spread a tiny little bit of the whipped butter on the tiny sliver of bread, she ate it. Oh, so good.

1/4 of the pretzel loaf … 115 calories
Smear of sweet butter … 65 calories

Time to order. Nikki looked around. People around her were shoveling bread and butter down their throats. The overweight lady next to her was being served a huge bowl of chicken alfredo. The gentleman across from her was having a slab of ribs and loaded baked potato. Thousands of calories. This empowered Nikki as she ordered her entrée from the Lite Fare Menu. She started with the Mediterranean salad with the dressing and feta on the side. For her course, she decided on the sea scallops. Her husband ordered the bang-bang shrimp for an appetizer and the blue cheese crusted filet for dinner. It never bothered her that he wasn't health conscious. She was so grateful that he was so supportive of her new lifestyle.

The salad arrived. They put the feta on the salad, but it didn't look like that much. Instead of sending it back, she just picked through it and tried not to eat all the cheese.

The dressing was in a tiny little cup. She first dipped her fork in the cup like you are supposed to. She then gently poured some of the dressing on the salad. By the time she was finished, she ended up using all the dressing and had eaten all the cheese. It wasn't that much ... She thought. She also ate one of her husband's shrimp appetizers. She didn't look those up, but everyone knows that shrimp are low in calories.

Mediterranean salad (without dressing or feta) ... 115 calories
dressing and feta ... 255 calories
one bang-bang shrimp ... 123 calories

Because Nikki was being calorie conscious, she told the waiter not to bring her glass of wine until dinner. She carefully nursed her vodka drink and made it last. She was so proud of herself. Normally by now she would have had two martinis and a glass of wine.

She heard Freddie Mercury from Queen singing in her head, "We are the champions … We are the champions …" as she patiently waited for her glass of cabernet sauvignon.

cabernet sauvignon, 8 ounces … 192 calories

Time for dinner. The lady next to her had devoured her platter of pasta. The gentleman across from her sat in front of his rack of rib bones waiting for his bill. Nikki was enjoying her evening and felt like a million bucks. In the past, she would have left this place with more than a thousand calories eaten … Her scallops were amazing. The portion was a bit small, but she realized it was from the lite menu, and she felt satisfied. She traded her husband a scallop for a piece of filet and a spoonful of garlic mashed potatoes. Nikki's taste buds tingled plenty as she tasted the butter from her husbands' dish. Delicious, but not worth it.

lite fare scallop dish ... 525 calories

bite of filet and potato ... 112 calories

The waiter asked Nikki if she wanted another glass of wine. Although she did, she turned it down. She needed to keep her calories within reason. She had run ten miles that morning, but she had eaten a hearty breakfast to fuel beforehand. After the run, she replenished her body by having a high-protein shake and lunch. She politely turned down the glass of wine and asked for the check.

She did it! The song in her head changed to "Celebration" by Kool & The Gang. We went from 1977 to 1980 with our song selection and then to a halting stop.

Champagne and chocolate-covered strawberries complimentary for the anniversary couple. Back to Queen we go ... "Another one bites the dust. Another one bites the dust. And another one gone, and another one gone. Another one bites the dust ..."

Motherfucker. She could feel the calculator tape tickling her shoulder as the gargoyles whipped their calculators back out.

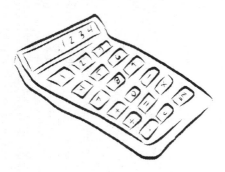

She was going to stay strong. Right away she took out her phone and looked up the calories of both the champagne and chocolate-covered strawberry. A standard glass of bubbly was 125 calories. A candied strawberry was 102. She knew she didn't want the entire thing but having half sounded amazing.

half of a chocolate-covered strawberry ...
51 calories

half of a glass of champagne ... 112.5 calories

Seriously? Have you ever had champagne
and chocolate-covered strawberries after
you have a full tummy? Give me a break.

the other half of a chocolate-covered
strawberry ... 51 calories

the other half of a glass of champagne ...
112.5 calories

Nikki initially felt guilty for her splurge,
but she knew it was well deserved. She also
knew that she stuck to her plan and did
relatively well. She thought about the lady
who ordered the pasta. That entrée was
more than 2,000 calories. Add the bread,
appetizers, and drinks. Nikki's calories were
a fraction of most others, and she felt great.

The next day Nikki decided she should
enter everything she had eaten into her food

log. She was very meticulous and included even the bites she took from her husband's plate. Since you have been previewing the entries as she consumed them, you may not be as shocked as she was. Here is a summary of what Nikki logged:

vodka water ... 105 calories

1/4 of the pretzel loaf ... 115 calories

smear of sweet butter ... 65 calories

Mediterranean salad ... 340 calories

one bang-bang shrimp ... 123 calories

cabernet sauvignon, 8 ounces ... 192 calories

lite fare scallop dish ... 525 calories

bite of filet and potato ... 112 calories

chocolate-covered strawberry ... 102 calories

glass of champagne ... 125 calories

grand total: 1,804 CALORIES

"Another one bites the dust. Another one bites the dust. And another one gone, and another one gone. Another one bites the dust."

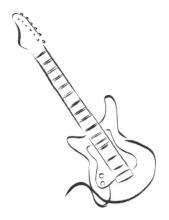

I realize how unfair this is.

It down right sucks.

This poor girl worked her ass off.

She did her homework.

She didn't order the drinks she wanted.

She didn't devour the bread.

She skipped the appetizer.

She had a freaking salad with barely any dressing on it.

For the love of God, she ordered the lowest calorie entrée off the stupid light menu.

It was so small too. She wanted to cry, but she didn't. She ate it like a big girl.

She watched everyone else shovel mashed fucking potatoes down their faces like it was feeding time at the zoo.

She didn't order the second glass of wine like everyone else at the Goddamn restaurant.

She was being good.

She didn't look at the freaking dessert menu and get to pick what looked good.

She ate a fucking piece of fruit with some chocolate on it for God's sake.

Could someone please turn the stupid music off in her head ... It was making her crazy.

It was just so unfair ...

Unfortunately, life doesn't have to be fair. It is what it is, and in this case, there was nothing that could be changed about this scenario. If Nikki had logged before she went to eat, she could have saved herself several hundreds of calories by illuminating a few things. The bottom line is that dining out puts you in a category of risk. Most people do not think about all the calories that are consumed when going out to eat. I'm not suggesting that you stop eating out completely, but I am telling you to be mindful of what you are doing. I am also saying that you should stop blaming your thyroid and hormones for your inability to lose weight and start paying attention to your actual caloric intake.

My clients who cannot lose weight are often guilty of eating out multiple times a week. I am unsure how accurate the calorie estimations of entrees are on menus. It is unclear to me how the portions of foods are measured in the chaos of the back kitchens. I am not implying that the eighteen-year-old food technicians aren't measuring the cheese they dump on your salad. However, I often wonder if the eighteen-year-old food technicians are measuring the cheese they dump on your salad.

Being mindless about what you're eating is one of the most dangerous behaviors you could develop. We have all sat and eaten stale popcorn and pizza that didn't taste great. We eat when we are on the phone. We eat when we are bored. We eat when we drive. When we don't pay attention to what we are eating, how much we are eating it becomes mindless. As explained earlier, if you didn't see it happen, then it didn't. That leads to denial. If you are wondering if the bite of steak and potato that Nikki sampled from her husband's dinner could really have been 112 calories, that isn't even a stretch. A buttery steak and potato entrée at a restaurant can be 2,000 calories or more. Yes, a hearty bite can easily be more than 100 calories. Let's think about how often we mindlessly take these bites and not count them.

There have been food studies done where people's behaviors are tested under different variables. One that I found interesting was conducted at a chicken wing restaurant. There was no limit to portions at this place on Tuesday night, as it's all-you-can-eat wing night. Time to feast. Clearly, the people dining here on Tuesdays are not watching their waistlines. Yet, it is still fascinating how the results of this experiment turned out.

The waitstaff was instructed to clear the table of the bones and wing debris after the patrons had finished a round of wings. They were asked to do this for only half the restaurant. This was group A. The other half of the tables had the waitstaff clear only soiled napkins off the table. This was group B. No other factors were changed. Both groups were asked for refills on drinks and wings equally throughout the night. At the end of the night, the number of chicken wings consumed were counted and compared. Group A consumed almost 30 percent more wings per person. This group had the bones cleared from the table, making the amount of food eaten less visible. As the group socialized, the wings disappeared, and the waitstaff replenished the plates with fresh batches. Once the remains were cleared away, there was no trace of what was done. Whether one, two, five, or twelve wings were eaten, no one really knew.

Group B, on the other hand, was faced with the remains of their feast. The waitresses left the remains in front of each person for them to see. The plates used in both groups were larger than usual to accommodate for the debris. As each person munched and finger licked, they made noticeable eye contact with the pile of bones.

Our stomach can't count, and we can't remember. Using our own perceived measure of fullness is not the best way to determine if we should stop eating. We are conditioned to finish all the food that is served to us. That is the expectation. Many households require their children to finish everything on their plate in order to get dessert. Dear Lord, this should be outlawed. Why do we force-feed our youth and force them to develop unhealthy eating habits? As a health-conscious parent, I never required my children to finish everything on their plates. Luckily for my children, I had this whole weight-loss thing figured out before I popped them out. This saved them the trouble of having to break the unnecessary bad habits that many Americans develop.

Globally, an estimated forty-three million children younger than five years of age were overweight in 2018—a 54 percent increase from 2000. Overweight and obese children are at higher risk of developing serious health problems, including type 2 diabetes and high blood pressure. Childhood obesity also increases the risk of obesity, noncommunicable diseases, premature death, and disability in adulthood.

It has been proven in multiple studies that parents who serve their children large portions are putting their kids at risk for adult obesity. Parents also play an important role in determining not only which foods but how much food children consume. It can often be difficult for many parents to assess appropriate portion sizes for children. They inadvertently contribute to the problem of overeating in children. Increasing single servings of commercially available foods may condition individuals into believing that larger portion sizes are normal. This may lead to overconsumption of those foods, but it can also be translated into larger portion sizes of home-prepared meals.

Learning to focus on internal cues of hunger and satiety will help us recognize when we are full. We should eat slowly and only when we are hungry. Using smaller sized serving bowls, utensils, and plates may also be effective at limiting the amount of food consumed. Having a large plate is like having a large purse. You know you're going to fill it with crap you don't need. If you use a small dinner plate, you will plan your portions better and most likely not go overboard. The last time I used a large tote bag I ended up fitting my entire dinner in it, along with a change of clothes. #fatpants #mindlesseating

Perceived Levels of Fullness

In addition to logging, it is important to walk away from the dinner table when you feel satisfied. This is a difficult task for most people, as they have been conditioned improperly by their parents or society. There are several charts available to show perceived hunger. I have developed my own. I council my clients to always identify what level they are in before, during, and after they are finished with each meal.

Level 0–2: Starving. You have not eaten in several hours. Your stomach is growling, and you are feeling weak and dizzy. You can feel that your blood sugar has dropped. You will eat pretty much anything. Moldy bread and expired lunchmeat don't seem to bother you.

Level 3–4: Hungry. Your last meal was three to four hours ago. You are feeling some hunger pangs. If you don't get food within the next twenty minutes, you will go bat-shit crazy on the next person who crosses your path. You need to eat something soon, or you may end up eating your shoe.

Level 5–6: Satisfied. You have just completed a meal. You feel satisfied but could also eat another helping. The amount of food that you have consumed is an adequate amount to provide enough energy for you to get through the next few hours. You know you should stop eating and are challenged to put the fork down.

Level 7–8: Full. The amount of food that you have consumed has exceeded the ideal amount that anyone should eat in one sitting. You feel like you have eaten far too much and need to loosen your top button. You regret eating so much and have called yourself a pig and a cow a few times. You know that in a few hours you won't feel this full and might want to eat again.

Level 9–10: Buffet stuffed. You have a stomachache and feel sick. You never want to eat again because you are at full capacity. If you sneeze or cough, you may vomit. You decide to go to bed early and hope the heartburn doesn't kill you before morning. You are definitely never eating again.

Okay, folks … I am starting to get tired. I'm thirteen chapters into this book. My brain hurts from explaining all this shit to you. I am 58,493 words into this masterpiece, and so are you. If you are going to make me explain which level of perceived hunger you should be in after you eat, I'm going to stab you with my fork. In the neck. Hard.

No need for violence.

Log your damn food.

Be mindful and true to yourself.

Don't be an askhole and ignore your behaviors.

The world is full of askholes.

It is my job that you do not become one.

Before we get into this very complicated topic, I need to get something to eat.

I'm suddenly craving peppermint mochas and chicken wings.

14

Askholes and Haters: Girlfriends Be Warned

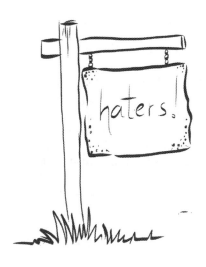

Ever since the beginning of time there have been haters. They come in all shapes and sizes. They can be young or old. They are miserable people who usually have miserable lives and shallow, empty, heartless souls with no regard for life. They often sit on lily pads and judge others as if their lives are perfect. These envious fuckers can be found anywhere in the world and in all walks of life. They hate. No matter what they say or pretend to be, deep inside their thick, evil skin is blood so cold that it makes them unable to have any compassion. They cannot have respect for other people's hard work and dedication.

These haters start out being little kid haters. They hate other little kids and make them cry. I remember Julie Lovelace in third grade. She was an evil little hating bitch bag that used to have a certain way with words. She could make grown men cry. I fucking hated that crotch. She has probably grown up to be a big-person hater who has tortured and destroyed hundreds of people in her life. She undoubtably has no understanding of the damage she has caused.

Once a hater grows up and becomes a skilled hater, I like to call them master haters. A master hater is someone who has moved up on the hater hierarchy. They are extremely skilled at hating and manipulating. Master haters are usually hard to spot. They are so skilled. They have an amazing ability to bullshit their way into your life and make you think they actually give a shit.

Why am I telling you this?

This is a book about weight loss, isn't it?

Take a quick minute and close this book. Don't lose this page, though, because then I won't be able to finish my point …

Look at the title of this book:

The Girlfriends' Guide to Weight Loss: What Your Doctors Can't Tell You and What Your Trainers Won't

Your doctors can't tell you about these haters. That is completely against their code of ethics. Your personal trainers won't tell you about them either. This would make them unprofessional and inappropriate. I am taking one for the team. I feel compelled to tell you that as you embark on this journey toward a healthier life, there are people in this world who are going to resent you for it. These people may be people who truly care about you—friends and relatives, coworkers and neighbors. They are going to appear to be supportive, so be warned. They are going to compliment you and help you as much as they can. You will be grateful for their support until one day when you see the hate thorns poking out of their heads.

I am unsure what happens to people, but it is an interesting phenomenon. As soon as you start losing weight and visibly looking different, people will try and derail you. It is not obvious at first. Some haters are very subtle with their suggestions to go out for lunch or bringing you cupcakes for no reason. I'm not even sure they realize they are trying to sabotage your efforts. It seems so innocent when they ask you to skip spin class to go out for brunch.

Slowly, these suggestions turn into backstabbing remarks. Often these comments are behind your back. They eventually surface to your face. Comments about always needing to eat healthy. Remarks about having to calculate calories of food. References to working out and being fit. Nonstop. At first, you will be flattered. Eventually, it will get old.

The issue here is that these haters cannot handle seeing you succeed. Most likely, they are unable to follow a plan and don't like seeing you thrive. These haters become vicious *crock-blocking* monsters after a certain time. A crock-blocker is someone who feeds you nonsense or a made-up story in order to prevent you from moving in the desired direction or path.

crock

/kräk/

something considered to be complete nonsense.

synonyms: lie, falsehood, fib, made-up story, invention, fabrication, deception, (piece of) fiction;

block·er

/'bläkər/

noun

a substance that prevents or inhibits a given physiological function. make the movement or flow in (a passage, pipe, road, etc.) difficult or impossible

synonyms: clog (up), stop up, choke, plug, obstruct, gum up, dam up, congest;

crock◆ block◆er

/kräk/ 'bläkər/

noun

a person who appears to be trying to help you but is actually trying to make it impossible for you to move toward your goal.

"Stefani was a crock-blocker when she told Mary that she thought she was getting too skinny, even though Mary still had a lot more weight to lose."

Synonyms: antagonist, opponent, enemy, rival;

I'm not suggesting that you go around thinking everyone is out to get you. I do want you to be aware of the target that will be on your butt as it starts looking better. The longer you stay on course, the more forward people will be. The comments will go from subtle to downright rude. You will be accused of being a diet cheater. You will be under speculation of taking diet shortcuts. You will be on the mean girls' text strings every time you leave the gym. It will happen. No matter how nice you are, people will want to dislike you for your success. They still love and respect you, but they will dislike you at the same time. There are some genuine people out there who won't try and derail you. They won't wish evil on you. They might, however, have secret wishes that you will gain back some of the weight you lost. They may fantasize about you skipping spin class for frickin' brunch just one of these days …

As I continue to talk about these crock-blockers, I have to point out that most of them do not know that they are being antagonizing—most of them. There are a handful of them who are perfectly aware of their asshole behavior. These haters are seasoned master-haters who do not want you to succeed. If they can't sabotage your success, they are crafty at making you question your goals. I have firsthand experience with these evil, cold-blooded behemoths, but I've had clients complain about them as well.

In fact, as soon as a client reaches his or her weight loss goal, that person inevitably asks my advice on this matter. This is a problem that occurs when people lose weight. I have seen these haters slither out of peoples' lives in all areas. Haters hate happy marriages. Haters hate successful careers. Haters hate people who make a lot of money. Haters hate because they are insecure. This is their problem, not yours. Since your doctors and trainers can't tell you this shit, I have to. I have seen successful people be taken down by loved ones. Sticks and stones can break your bones. Although words could never hurt you, they do.

Here are some of the more hurtful remarks I have heard over the years. I am including some strategies to help cope with these remarks. Remember, people who go out of their way to make you feel inferior need to self-reflect. They are like bullfrogs, sluggish and miserable, sitting on their lily pads judging everyone else but not seeing their own shortcomings. Just like the bullfrog in chapter 5 that no one liked. They are most likely the ones who need to help themselves. #hatersgonnahate #bullfrogsarestupid

Popular Hater Comments That You Should Not Let Bother You

+ Aren't you tired of not eating real food?
+ What's going to happen when you get tired of working out every day?
+ Does your husband get mad that you go to the gym after work?
+ My kids would never let me serve food like that.
+ I could never spend money on a gym membership.
+ You get up at four o'clock in the morning? Don't you feel bad when you fall asleep and your kids are still awake at night?
+ Your knees are going to end up needing replacements.
+ Isn't it bad to work out every day?
+ I heard that you shouldn't drink so much water. Why are you drinking so much water?
+ Your knees are going to end up needing replacements.

+ I would feel like such a bad mom if I left my kids to go running in the morning.

+ I could never cook that way. It is way too expensive.

+ You spend too much time on yourself.

+ My husband would get angry if I had to buy new clothes.

+ Don't you feel bad that you spend so much time on this weight-loss thing? I would feel guilty.

+ You are starting to look too skinny.

+ How much more weight are you going to lose?

+ Your face is looking gaunt.

+ Your knees ...

+ I heard it is bad for your heart to do cardio every day. Have you told your doctor?

+ I heard you can get kidney stones if you eat all that protein.

+ My kids would never let me spend so much time on myself. I would feel like I was neglecting them.

+ Your knees ...

+ I think you have lost enough weight.

+ My neighbor's sister's cousin's friend's ex-boyfriend's roommate said that people who lose weight end up getting divorced.

+ I think you looked really good when you lost the first ten pounds.

+ I made cookies, but you probably won't eat one so I didn't bring you one.

+ You're not the same as you were before you lost weight.

+ Your knees …

Wow. I could spend all day generating more of these. Looking back at them all, every single one is bullshit. Bullshit is for bullfrogs. Clearly, these remarks stem from jealousy and insecurity. You should not let anyone derail you. Don't let anyone make you feel bad for spending time on yourself. Some people spend time getting their nails done. Some go to the spa for hours or spend hours golfing with their friends. You are entitled to go for a run. Don't let them make you feel bad about that.

You are being a role model to your children by reaching a goal that you have set for yourself. You are getting stronger and feeling better. These things are all making you a better wife and mother. They are making you a better friend and neighbor. All of this exercise is strengthening your heart and even your knees. You could lash back with a rude comment to any of these illogical statements. You don't need to because the way you look and feel is painful enough for these haters to see. Smile and know that they have noticed how amazing you look in your new wardrobe. You are doing this for you!

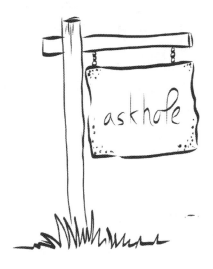

There are haters, and there also are askholes. Askholes are not as vicious as haters, mostly because they usually have a much lower IQ. They can't help it that they are stupid. They were born that way. They are too dumb to know the difference and have no ability to fix it. An askhole is a person who truly wants your advice. They ask for it but then refuse to do to what you have to say. They end up doing things their own stupid way, despite the fact that you wasted your time giving them advice.

Askholes are usually very stubborn people who like to hear themselves talk. They are people who think they know more than you and everyone else in the world, including God. Askholes are an interesting breed of people. They shouldn't have friends, but somehow they do. This means they are either lying or these friends don't actually exist.

Askholes tend to surface anytime the topic of losing weight comes up. These persistent souls will beat you down until they get you to tell them exactly what you did to lose weight. They want to hear it all—every single detail—but they need you to explain it in five minutes or less. They are listening to everything you are saying because they are planning on going home and duplicating your exact routine. As you speak, you are quickly interrupted. An askhole will interrupt you frequently to interject her version of what should be done. She will throw in irrelevant information that has nothing to do with what she asked you about. Usually within minutes, the askhole has monopolized the conversation and is now telling you how to lose weight.

I'm warning you. This will happen. It happens to me, and I have twenty years' experience and certificates to validate my research. I somehow always find myself nodding my head politely—nodding and smiling as I pretend to scribble the word *askhole* on the person's forehead with a purple crayon.

What happens on the rare occasion that you come across someone evil enough yet stupid enough to be a hater and askhole combined? This is a very unique combination. Yet, this selfish bitch-bag of a moron exists. I need to warn you. You need to watch for them. You may not have encountered them yet. As soon as you start losing weight, these fuckers start showing up every Goddamn place that you're at. Parties, bus stops, picnics, garage sales, grocery stores, you name it. Haters and askholes. Flocked like bullfrogs in a pond. All over the fucking place, just hating every inch of you for no reason. Wanting to know exactly what your secrets are. Telling you things that are false and untrue. Myths. Fallacies. #goddamnbullfrogs #hatersgonnahate #karmaisabitch

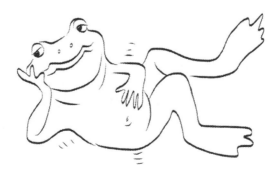

Girlfriends be warned, there are so many. Your doctors won't tell you about these either. Your trainers may actually think they are true. All I know is thank goodness for me and my willingness to write this book. I really am the best....

15

Myth Busters:
The Fallacies of Fitness

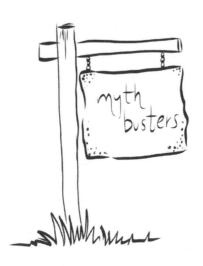

s it true? There are many, many ridiculous myths in the fitness and nutrition world. Many have been around for decades. Although fitness fables are jacked up, some have some logical reasoning. This makes everything so much more confusing than it needs to be. I often wonder where these tales came from. Did someone deliberately release them into the world, like a flock of birds? Perhaps the askholes who hide behind locker room stalls at the gym overhear information and add their own two cents to the fact. The fact has now become askhole hogwash. It's like playing the telephone game but with nutritional information.

You remember the telephone game. I'll never forget playing it at slumber parties. One time the original message was: "My favorite thing to do is go to the pool and pick up hot guys." After one rotation around the room, it quickly turned to: "My favorite kind of food is pickled poop and hot fries." Imagine how funny this was to a bunch of twelve-year-old girls. I actually think this would be a fun game to play now with a side of vodka on a girls' night out, but I would have to stay up past my bedtime for that, and we all know *that's* not happening.

Back to my point. Information often is miscommunicated from person to person and becomes invalid. People may put their own twist to things and pass on their version of the fact.

This fact has now become a myth. There are many of these myths in existence. Some are related to fitness; many are not. Urban legends. Many of these legends are so arguably true that people have written books about their validity. Over the years, I have found myself spending countless hours researching certain tales myself. Initially, I fell into the trap of believing these tales were true. After I slapped myself in the face a few times and realized I was being an ass, I looked this shit up. Sure enough, I was being misled—another inspiration for me to write this book. #thankgoodnessforme

The urban legend that I believed for years led to an interesting study that I conducted with a group of clients. We have all heard that you shouldn't eat past seven o'clock in the evening if you are trying to lose weight. They say that if you eat that close to bed, all of the calories that you consume sit in your stomach and don't digest while you are sleeping. The calories will all turn to fat faster, and it is harder to lose the weight. They say this will happen. Once again, who the hell is *they*? I feel as if *they* is like the Wizard of Oz—this invisible being who dictates all these facts but has absolutely no proof that the information is valid. No one argues with "they" because they are they. Just like no one would dare argue with Oz.

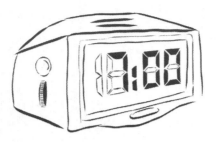

Let's go back and reread the eating past seven o'clock myth.

"If you eat past seven o'clock at night, all of the calories you consume will sit in your stomach and not digest. These calories will all turn to fat faster, and it will be harder to lose the weight."

Is it just me, or does that not sound ridiculous when you actually read it and break it down? If you are scratching you head wondering what you are missing, I will explain it to you. You are still in kindergarten, so I cannot judge.

1. Your body does not know what time it is. It can't tell if it is three o'clock or seven o'clock. This is like watering a plant. If the plant needs water, it doesn't matter if you water it at five o'clock or eight o'clock. When you water the plant, the soil will absorb the water. It does not matter what time you water the

plant. If the plant needs to be watered, then it does not matter what time you water it, just as long as you water it.

2. Your body burns calories at the same rate whether the sun is shining or it's bedtime. There is no research that indicates that people burn fewer calories at night or during the day. If you have not reached your caloric limit for the day, you can eat even if it is at midnight. Let's suppose you have a 1,500 calorie allowance for the day, and you have 600 calories left for dinner. If you eat that 600-calorie dinner at five o'clock, your body will absorb the nutrients and burn the calories as needed for the remainder of the day. What does not get burnt on that day will the following day or be stored as fat. If you don't eat your 600-calorie dinner until nine o'clock, the same exact thing will occur. It does not matter what time you eat just as long as you don't go over your calorie allowance. That is the key. Most people who eat past a certain hour end up overeating because they can't stop. They mindlessly stuff their faces without paying attention to the quantity of calories that they are consuming.

3.   Calories will not turn to fat faster if you eat past a
     certain hour. Read that again. Calories will not turn
     to any faster after seven o'clock. If that is not the
     most asinine thing you have ever heard of, I don't
     know what is. Why on earth would a calorie turn
     to fat faster after seven? It's not a fucking pumpkin,
     and it's not midnight. First of all, calories don't turn
     into fat. Calories measure energy. They will not turn
     into fat. Even if they did, it would make no sense to
     assume that the time of day would matter. When
     you consume calories, your body has to burn them.
     What doesn't get burned that day will get stored
     and burned the following day. If you are in a caloric
     deficit, your body will burn your fat stores for energy.
     In order to lose weight, you need to put yourself into a
     caloric deficit. The deficit should be the total number
     of calories overall. Overall, not daily. You see, your
     body doesn't end each day like your log does. Your
     body sees the big picture: total number of calories
     consumed versus total number of calories expended.
     If you eat a meal past a certain hour and you are in a
     caloric deficit, you still will lose weight. Once again,
     it is not like your body understands time. You're not

at the movie theater where the prices go up after a certain time. Seriously, people.

4. The calories you consume will digest, and they won't just sit in your stomach. This cracks me up. I have this visual of someone eating a late dinner and thinking that the food is going to sit in her gut all night. Do people really think that our digestive systems turn off when we go to sleep? If this were true, then everything we ate would actually rot in our stomachs as we slept for the eight hours. We would wake up with rancid odors seeping from our bodies because the food we ate would be sitting idle for hours. We would wake up feeling sick and unable to eat because we would still have undigested food in our systems from the night before. Our digestive systems are constantly working. No matter what time it is, if you swallow something, your stomach is ready to receive it and process it. It will process it the same way at five o'clock in the morning as it will at midnight.

To answer the question, it is *not true* that eating past seven o'clock at night (or any hour) can cause weight gain. There is no research, study, or individual who has ever gained weight simply by eating past a certain hour. However, be warned because people who eat past a certain hour do have a higher chance of gaining weight. Are you confused? Let me explain.

There was a study done in which one hundred people were told not to eat past seven o'clock for one month, group A. Their behaviors were studied and watched. The participants were asked to log everything they ate throughout the day and up until their seven o'clock deadline. These individuals were generally healthy eaters. In the study, a second group of one hundred people were also watched, group B. They were also healthy eaters and were told to log everything they ate. They had no deadline by which they had to stop eating.

It was concluded that people in group A lost weight only because they did not go over their caloric limit. They were placed under a restriction of not eating past a certain hour, which caused them to not eat. This had nothing to do with consuming calories past that hour.

Group B, on the other hand, spent several hours after dinner mindlessly eating. The average amount of calories consumed after dinner was 655 calories each night. This is the overall average amount of calories consumed over the month. The average dinner time was six o'clock in the evening. The average bedtime was ten thirty. The four and a half hours that people had in between dinner and bedtime was spent grazing on food. Handfuls of nuts, chips, and ice cream. Alcoholic beverages were a contributing factor as well. In conclusion, it was determined that creating an eating deadline could cause someone to lose weight. The time of day had nothing to do with it.

This is just one example of a myth that exists in the world of fitness and nutrition. I don't want you to fall into the trap of any of the others. I caution you to always be warned when you hear the words "they say" or "I heard." These are red flags that an askhole made up this tale, and you should be warned. Here are a few more of my favorites:

Negative calorie foods help you burn calories.

A little bullfrog may have told you to munch on celery or iceberg lettuce because digesting these veggies burns more calories than the actual vegetable provides—but do you actually believe the hype? The urban myth around so-called negative-calorie foods is based on an actual proven scientific effect, known as the thermic effect of food, which ranges in percentage from 10 to 20 percent concerning the amount of energy expended by the body to digest any given food. So, if the thermic effect of food maxes out at 20 percent, you can only, realistically, burn 20 percent of the total caloric value of any food you eat. That means the idea that digesting food could put you at a deficit as far as caloric intake is illogical.

Fat turns to muscle, or muscle turns to fat.

Muscle and fat are made up of entirely different types of tissues. One cannot transform into the other. That would be like saying your bread turned to butter. It can't happen. If you stop working out, your muscle mass will decrease. If you start eating bad, your body fat will increase. One will not transform into another. If your personal trainer is telling you that they can turn the flab off your arms into a sculpted muscle, then you need to find a new one. Unless they are a magician, it's not happening.

Juice cleanses work.

Superstar Beyoncé was reputed to sip 600-calorie-per-day diets consisting of lemon-infused water with maple syrup and cayenne pepper on the advice of fitness gurus in order to shed pounds. It's no wonder why many North Americans think a juice cleanse is the only way to detox and lose weight successfully. The idea behind a juice cleanse is to give your gastrointestinal tract a break from solid food by using liquids to flush toxic sludge from your body and speed up metabolism.

Americans think that doing these cleanses is a quick way to lose weight. It's easier than figuring out what to eat. You don't have to cook. You can just torture yourself for a week and drop several pounds. It's great! The problem is that it is impossible to maintain. Let's be real, people! We need food. We need to chew. There is nothing wrong with making a flipping salad and eating it. Why throw spinach, kale, apple, cucumber, celery, and carrots in the blender and choke it down? I'd much rather dice up the spinach and kale, cube up the carrots and celery, dice up the cucumber and apple, squeeze the lemon on top, and eat it with a fork.

I realize the purpose of juicing is to give your body a break from digesting, but let's be real. How many people finish these detoxes and dive into a bag of potato chips the size of Nebraska. If you are going to detox, then do it for the right reasons. #nopizzaforyou

It takes twenty-one days to break bad habits and establish good ones.

The perplexing thing about being human is that we are all unique individuals. There is no miracle time frame that can be attributed to establishing healthy habits and breaking bad ones. Our bodies do not have a special clock built in that goes off after twenty-one days that alerts us that a habit is broken or formed. People face challenges, establish new routine, and withstand temptation differently. Time duration widely differs, and no magical one-size-fits-all time frame can be applied to creating new habits and breaking bad habits. If someone is able to break a bad habit sooner than the three-week time frame, being told that it takes longer can serve as a distraction.

Coffee is bad for you.

I was relieved to finally uncover the truth behind this myth. Although I am not a huge coffee drinker, I do enjoy my coffee. Despite the fact that java is rich in caffeine, a cup of coffee actually holds many health benefits. Firstly, coffee is a rich source of cancer-blasting antioxidants. It has been found that regular coffee sipping reduced the rates of Alzheimer's and Parkinson's disease, type 2 diabetes, and depression, linking the magical brew to extended longevity. As long as you hold the whip and don't load up on cream and sugar, it won't affect your waistline.

Sea salt is better than table salt.

Regardless what they say, both contain the same amount of sodium (roughly 2,300 milligrams per tablespoon). Table salt contains iodine, whereas sea salt does not. The sea salt may add a lot brinier flavor, resulting in less salt use overall, but neither type of salt contains enough of any one beneficial mineral to make it the healthier option. Himalayan pink rock salt has become a popular trend. It's still salt. Use it sparingly. If you put it all over your french fries, it won't magically make your fries healthy.

Eggs are bad for you because of the cholesterol.

Debunked! For years, eggs have gotten the bad rap for causing high cholesterol in people. Recently, it has been proven that the cholesterol in the diet doesn't really raise the cholesterol in blood. In fact, eggs primarily raise the good cholesterol and are *not* associated with increased risk of heart disease. Eggs are, in fact, one of the most nutritious foods available! They're high in all sorts of nutrients, along with unique antioxidants that protect our eyes. To top it all off, despite being a high-fat food, eating eggs for breakfast is proven to cause weight loss.

Carbs are bad for you.

Carbs are not bad for you. Even too many carbs aren't necessarily bad for you. What people are trying to say is that too many carbs can cause someone to gain weight. That is more accurate. Dr. Atkins developed the Atkins diet, which gained popularity in the early 2000s. This also caused Americans to have a somewhat distorted way of thinking when it comes to carbohydrates. If you have ever done the Atkins diet, you are told to avoid all carbs. You are limited to 20 grams each day. This is an impossibly low amount of carbohydrates.

The point of this is to get your body into ketosis, which will cause it to burn fat for fuel. It really does work. The issue is the sustainability of this program. Twenty grams of carbs in a full day means no fruit, no grains, and no starches. It means no bread, no carrots, no tomatoes, and no fun. With all this being said, carbs still are not bad for you. Dr. Atkins did create a fear of carbs in our society. People think they will make you gain weight. In reality, carbohydrates need to be part of your diet. Moderation is the key. Too many carbs will cause you to gain weight. Learning the right amount that you should eat is essential. I laugh when clients are afraid to put corn on their salads because it's a carb. Yet, they will mindlessly eats a bag of potato chips while making the salad.

You should work out on an empty stomach.

During cardio, performance and energy expenditure in the fasted state are about the same as in fed state. In the fasted state, you'll burn more body fat, but that won't make it easier for you to use body fat as fuel during the rest of the day (when you're fed). You'll also burn a tiny bit more muscle, but you'll grow it back faster afterward too. It seems to balance out (as long as you get enough protein). Finally, cardio suppresses appetite less in the fasted state than in the fed state, but that doesn't translate into a significant difference in daily caloric intake. Basically, in the end, it is the same; therefore, it is a matter of personal preference.

You should eat protein immediately after you work out.

When you exercise, you damage your muscles. Your body then needs to repair. This makes them more resilient in the process. The raw material for this repair is the protein you ingest. You need protein right after your workout may not be a myth so much as an exaggeration. Consuming

20–40 grams of protein within the two hours following your workout may be ideal, but it isn't necessary. What matters most is your total daily protein intake. Don't be fooled into thinking you need to cram it in all at once.

Cardio machines give you accurate readings.

Don't believe the screen. There is no way any device can give you the exact amount of calories burned. There is no watch, treadmill, elliptical, or app that can give you this number. The amount of calories burned are calculated by a program that uses your weight and your heart rate to come up with what you burned. It gives an approximate number. This can be close to the actual amount, or it can be off by a landslide. The longer you stay on the machine, the greater the line of error will be. If you are on the treadmill for fifteen minutes and it says you burnt 150 calories when you only burnt 110, then there isn't that much of a difference. If you were on the treadmill for two hours and you were told you burned 1,100 calories when you only burnt 611, then that could be an issue. Don't believe the screen.

Sit-ups will get you a six-pack.

Although doing abdominal exercises will help tone your tummy, it is not the only way to get that chiseled six-pack. You can do sit-ups all day long, but if you don't watch what you put in your mouth, that six-pack will never shine. Strengthening your core involves doing exercises that include more than just regular sit-ups. Cardio is needed in order to trim the fat off your belly, along with whole body conditioning to develop strong muscles. Everyone has a six-pack; it just has to be uncovered a bit, and sit-ups are not the only way to do it.

You shouldn't do the same workout twice in a row.

I have heard this so many times over the years I could pull my hair out. It's a misconception that you shouldn't do the same exact workout every single day for a straight month … or year. You can, however, do similar workouts daily, and that will not hurt you. Runners who run every day don't have issues with their muscles getting confused. Swimmers swim daily and need to in order to build the strength and endurance required for their sport. Bikers spend hours on their bikes biking miles and miles every day so they can prepare for distance rides. You can work the same body part two or three days in a row. It will not confuse your body. If you start feeling pain or feel you are injured from the repetition of the movement, then that is a different story. Taking a weight listing class or doing a circuit where you are doing bicep work every day will not compromise your health in any way.

Lifting weights will make you bulky.

Again, another hair-pulling statement. I have a muscular frame. In my twenties, I was pretty muscular. I hated when people asked me if I was a bodybuilder. My arms were still much smaller than most, measuring at 9 inches. I still had people tell me they didn't want to lift weights because it would make them become too bulky. Listen, you cannot lift a weight that is too heavy for you to lift. Right? At least I can't. If you do lift a very heavy weight, you can lift it all day long, and it will not make your muscles miraculously grow.

I picture the Incredible Hulk busting through his clothes as he gets angry. You would have to work really hard by adding a tremendous amount of protein and vigorous weight training into your schedule to get muscles like the Hulk. A regular strength training routine will not do that. Also, your fat cannot turn to muscle, remember.

Cycling and running will make your butt big.

I swear people who dislike exercise have made these up. Running and cycling are the two things that helped trim my thunder thighs down. I was known as elephant legs in high school and was teased and bullied as a freshman for my tree trunk stumps. I thought nothing could trim them down. I then started cycling and running. I'm not going to lie. I fell into the trap of thinking my thunder thighs were going to become rumbling thunder thighs when I started. That's what they said.

Too much cardio is bad for your heart.

Obviously, too much of anything is not good for anyone. If you are spending hours upon hours on the treadmill every day, I would question more than just the welfare of your heart. There is no research that indicates that excessive cardio is harmful to your heart. Endurance athletes have been researched and studied for years. There are some cases in which excessive exercise can affect the pathways of the heart in ultramarathon runners. Other studies show enlarged hearts in athletes due to the hours spent exercising. The population of people who fall into this category is less than 1 percent, and I am guessing if this were you that you would most likely be in such great shape that you and your doctor would be aware of your activity.

I once had a 280-pound client ask me if I was worried that all of my running was going to eventually kill me. I'll never forget looking at her. She still had the imprints on her face from the sleep apnea mask. I wanted so badly to ask her if it made her feel better about her poor health habits to draw attention to matters that didn't concern her. I decided to be the better person and ignore her ignorant comment. She was stupid anyway and ended up being the biggest askhole I ever met. #dontbeahater

Eating several small meals is better than eating three large meals.

It's easy to trace this myth back to its origin. Digestion does raise your metabolism a little, so eating less food and more often should keep your metabolism elevated, in theory. In practice, evidence shows that, given an equal number of daily calories, the number of meals largely makes no difference in fat loss.

Moreover, some studies suggest that having smaller meals more often makes it harder to feel full, potentially leading to increased food intake. Your metabolism can fluctuate based on the size of the meal, so fewer but larger meals means a larger spike in metabolism. Over the course of a day or week, given an equal number of calories, the number of meals doesn't seem to matter. It all evens out.

Fasting for several hours is good for your metabolism.

When you dramatically reduce your calorie intake, you will lose weight. It can also cause all kinds of health problems, including muscle loss. Further, when you start fasting, your body goes into conservation mode, burning calories more slowly. Keep in mind that the initial weight lost on a fast is primarily fluid or water weight, not fat. And when you go back to eating, any lost weight usually gets a return ticket back. Not only do most people regain weight lost on a fast, but they tend to add a few extra pounds because a slower metabolism makes it easier to gain weight. Worse, the weight that is regained is likely to be all fat. Lost muscle has to be added back at the gym. Nutrition experts agree that fasting is a potentially dangerous and not a particularly effective way to lose weight. Furthermore, there is no proof that it is good for your metabolism in any way. It is a trend, and it is a buzzword. Eat the way you are supposed to.

I can go on forever, but I won't. I have much better things to do with my time than yap about all the hogwash people hear about. Although a lot of the myths listed above are very believable, most of them can be debunked with a little internet research. It doesn't take a lot of time or knowledge to look up information and get the facts straight. Listening to false information can be very misleading. Always remember that telephone game, and don't forget how things can be misinterpreted. Be careful where you read your facts, as not all information may be validated.

16

Trust the Process: Believe and You Shall Receive

Trust the process. Trust the process. Trust the process. Trust the process. Trust the process.

Trust the process. Trust the process. Trust the process. Trust the process. Trust the process.

No matter how it's written, it is the most important thing you can say to yourself. You do not need to like the way the process works. You do not need to fully understand it. You don't even need to agree with it. You just have to trust it.

What exactly is this process that I speak of?

It's the meticulous process of losing weight. It's the tedious, gut-wrenching process of watching your body not cooperate the way you want it to. It's the awful undertaking of losing body fat that takes a thousand times longer than you think it should. It's the series of events that will take you much longer than anticipated—the events that will also drain and consume you for days and weeks until you become so frustrated that you want to quit.

This process is one that has its own mind. It's like a monster that has been possessed by the devil. You can't control it, and it can't control itself. It is unpredictable and unreliable. You can't punish it for being a jackass because you need it to cooperate. It has you by the balls, even when you don't have balls. It kicks you and makes you wish you could kick back. Yet you can't because you have to trust it. The motherfucking process. You need it because you know it works. It may be an asshole, but it works. It will only work if you trust it. If you don't believe in it, then it is useless. Having faith in the process will cause it to blossom and grow. It's like Christmas. Believe, and you shall receive.

Believe. Believe in the process. Believe in the series and steps that need to be taken in order to achieve a particular goal.

The process of losing weight is one that is very unpredictable. This is what makes this one so frustrating. People like to plan. People like things to fall into place like puzzle pieces. We like being told what our expectations should be along the way. These timelines help us get through life.

I thought of writing a book titled *What to Expect When You're Expecting to Lose Weight.* I decided that was impossible because no two people share the same experience. Although we all experience similar adventures throughout the way, there is no clear-cut expectation. You won't lose one or two pounds a week every single week like the books say you will. You will not see a one-pound loss on the scale for every 3,500-calorie deficit you create. It is not as simple as calories in versus calories out. These things will all frustrate you. They will derail you and make you want to quit. Many of you have quit before as a result of this. You feel cheated on. You are mad. You don't understand how you can work so hard at something and see no result.

Who are you mad at?

The process.

You're mad that you have devoted hours meal prepping on the weekends. Upset that you have packed your meals every day and brought food to work in fancy little containers.

You're livid that you skipped lunch dates with friends many times. You have woken up early to work out and stayed up late to get your steps in. You have counted calories and logged your food. Drank your water and skipped your wine. You have committed yourself to this, just like you always do, and after a whole month, you don't see that much of a result.

You are pissed. You are so mad that you decide you are going to get back at the process. Most people like to get their revenge by punishing the process. This is typically how this goes ...

Jenna was an overachiever. She was used to everything being planned out perfectly and executed as planned. When she started her diet, she got her calendar out and highlighted the dates that she would cross certain weight milestones. She was certain that everything would go as planned because she was going to do everything right. There was not going to be any cheating. There were not going to be any modifications made. Jenna was going to nail this and meet her weight-loss goal not a day later than planned.

At the beginning, everything went as planned. She was even ahead of schedule as she was losing more than just a few pounds a week at first. Jenna was feeling amazing. She knew she would be able to maintain this program and meet her goals. She was loving this new lifestyle and felt great.

One morning Jenna woke up to weigh herself and the scale showed that she gained 0.8 pounds. Although she knew that this slight weight gain could just be a weight fluctuation, she reweighed herself seventeen times to be sure. Jenna had to accept that she was up in weight for some reason, and she was not going to let it ruin her day. Although it did …

She texted her life coach to tell her the annoying news. Jenna's coach explained to her that there will be weight fluctuations and that she couldn't expect to see a loss every day. Jenna understood this but was still frustrated. The next day when she weighed she was down a full pound. The 0.8 lost along with an additional 0.2, making Jenna very happy.

This pattern continued for days and weeks until finally one day the scale did the unthinkable. It got stuck. The scale did not move for several days. Keep in mind that Jenna had lost more than ten pounds in less than a month—a bumpy ride down, but definitely down. Now it had been almost a straight week, and the scale had not moved an ounce. Jenna had not changed a thing. She was still following the program exactly as she should be. The first few days the scale didn't move she was able to accept that and continue on. There was definitely a dark shadow over those days, but she kept plugging along like a trooper.

Then, at almost a week, Jenna was downright mad. She sought revenge. She was angry, and everyone who had ever annoyed her was going to get it. First things first, her askhole neighbor Maddie. This know-it-all thought organic canned beans were healthier than fresh ones and drinking preworkout shakes made you burn more calories. Jenna had wanted to throat punch her the day she met her in spin class one day when she showed up with her boobs hanging out and acting like she knew more than the instructor.

Next, her husband. He was going to get it. She was tired of him leaving a trail of shit wherever he went. Why couldn't he just put his crap away like everyone else? His balls were getting served on a platter for dinner all because the scale hadn't moved. Poor guy.

The went goes on. Jenna had some rage brewing in her veins, and she was going to explode. Organic beans, boobs, and husband balls. She was pissed at the world.

In addition to her internal rage, Jenna felt the need to punish the food plan that she was on. She was very upset that it was not working the way it should. She was mad that it was not doing its job. Just like her husband who didn't pick up after himself, the food plan needed to be punished. Like Maddie who needed to be kicked in the crotch, the diet needed a slap. On the fifth day of seeing no loss, Jenna was making her kids breakfast. To her unexpected surprise, she started eating part of her son's waffle.

Holy crap. The crisp, warm waffle with the creamy butter dripping off the ends.

The maple syrup.

So sweet.

She didn't remember syrup tasting that sweet before. In fact, she never really liked waffles. Why was this so amazing?

It didn't matter because she was going to treat herself and have a waffle. Or three.

Five waffles later, Jenna felt self-defeated. She not only ate five waffles but also missed spin class because of her breakfast binge. As she sat at the kitchen table and scrolled through Facebook, she managed to come up with all sorts of fun dinner recipes that she was going to enjoy that were not on the plan. She was going to do some damage.

Jenna happened to come across a post of Maddie McBoobs in the spin class that she'd missed that morning. That fueled the fire even more, and now Jenna was going to do some serious damage. Maddie McBoobs ... Damn her.

Jenna had a feast that lasted for two days. She ate everything that she had been craving over the last month: chips, pizza, Chinese, pasta, burgers, bacon ... You name it. Jenna ate it. She felt accomplished, as she was teaching her diet a lesson. She was showing it how angry she was. No one could mess with her. No one.

A few days later when Jenna came to her senses, she had to face the music. She was bloated. Her stomach hurt. Nothing tasted good. She had no appetite. She had no energy and was always tired. She didn't want to admit that her plan to punish her diet had backfired and that she was being punished. Jenna was stubborn, and she was going not going to go down without a fight. She stripped down and hopped on the scale. She was not surprised to see that she had gained four pounds as a result of her revenge. Jenna knew that most of this gain was temporary and would drop relatively quickly, as she was retaining water from her recent binge.

After a week, Jenna was happy to be back to her prebinge weight. Looking at her calendar, she had wasted more than two weeks trying to teach this nonexistent thing a lesson. Unlike her husband or Maddie McBoobs, Jenna couldn't just take her frustrations out by having a confrontation or argument. The only one who suffered here was her. Jenna suffered, and her metabolism suffered.

Luckily, Jenna had an amazing life coach who encouraged her to get back on track. Normally, Jenna would have quit. Historically, Jenna had given up at this point. Usually, she threw in the towel right about now—right about the time when she was trying to teach the process a lesson.

Her life coach had changed her mind-set. Her coach told her that she needed to trust the process. She needed to learn to believe in the process, much like believing in Santa. The second you start having doubts, you lose the confidence needed to persevere. Because you cannot control what your body is going to do and how your body is going to react, you just have to have faith. You have to have faith that following the plan and doing everything right will eventually bring you the results that you are working for. There is no way that your goals will not be met if you stick to the plan. At that point, Jenna's life coach asked her to repeat the following statement:

"If I am doing everything right and the scale isn't moving, I have shouldn't stress. The scale will eventually move, and I have nothing to worry about. There is more to this lifestyle than just the numbers on the scale. I feel great, and I will keep moving strong."

Jenna repeated this over and over. She repeated this on days that the scale didn't cooperate. She chanted this when she wanted to quit. She also started to trust the process. Jenna realized that this whole process was indeed a process. It was one that was not cut and dry. It wasn't black-and-white. It couldn't be planned out precisely and figured out perfectly. It was stubborn, like a three-year-old who will fight you until he wins. Like a husband who won't listen time after time to your requests to pick up his damn socks.

There are some things in life you can't control, and you have to deal with. Like Maddie's boobs bouncing away in spin class week after week. You don't have to like them, but they are there, and you have to deal with them. You also don't have to like that the scale may not move for several days or weeks. Unfortunately, your choice is to be patient and continue working hard or jump ship and eat your weight in waffles.

Trust the process. Trust that it will pay off. Know that it is a slow and unpredictable undertaking. If you resist it, then it will prolong things. If you question it, you will be consumed with frustration. If you try to change it, you will find that it can't be modified. You either have to learn to trust it, or it will destroy you. I realize you are only in kindergarten. Up until now I have asked you to keep everything basic. Now, at the very end of the very last chapter, I ask you to do the most complex thing ever. Trust the process. How can you trust something that you don't understand? You must have faith … You must be patient.

You must have faith that this process will work, and you must have patience. Not only do you have to reach your goal, but then you have to maintain it. I'm pretty sure you already know this, but once you reach your goal, you have to continue working in order to retain the results you have achieved. I have mentioned this several times, but statistically, people have a 5 percent chance of keeping the weight they have lost off unless they lose it the right way. The right way: a realistic and sustainable program that allows you to indulge and teaches you to self-forgive, a program that bases its curriculum on being patient and understanding that this process will come with mistakes and should lifelong.

I have seen the pounds pack back on many of my clients over the years. I have seen the pounds pack on myself as well, and I will not have it anymore. Maintenance does not need to be difficult. Stay on track. Continue applying the behaviors that you implemented when you lost the weight, and you will have no problem. This is no different than anything else in life …

Meet Billy Jean.

Billy Jean always wanted a beautifully landscaped house. Every time she tried to clean up her flower beds and bushes, it would never last. One day Billy Jean decided she was going to devote herself to accomplishing this goal.

She spent *months* pulling weeds, trimming trees, fertilizing, planting, and taking care of her garden.

She worked every single day … day in and day out. She thought about it nonstop and educated herself on how to take care and maintain this beautiful garden. She devoted her heart and soul into this. She made sure to fit it into her routine without compromising all of the other important things in her life. There were some days when Billy Jean didn't feel like trimming the trees, so she would skip a day here and there. She always felt icky on those days and would get back to her gardening.

One time she took an entire week off for a trip. She had extra weeds to pull and fertilizing to do when she returned.

She did it, and the garden looked beautiful. In years past, Billy Jean would go on vacation and just let her garden go right back to where it started. Weeds, dead flowers, and even a bunch of garbage would pile up. Not this time. She came back from the trip and gave her garden some TLC, and *bam*. She knew that starting over and making her garden beautiful again was *far more* work than just maintaining it.

At first, no one noticed Billy Jean's garden was looking better. This would frustrate her. She could see the difference, and that was very motivating. She often looked at the other beautiful gardens in her neighborhood. That was her inspiration.

Once people started noticing, Billy Jean was constantly being asked how she was able to make her garden look so good. People wanted Billy Jean to say she hired someone or sprinkled some magical powder around her home. Billy Jean would tell people how she completely changed her routine and made her garden her priority. No shortcuts. Just hard work. She was now the inspiration.

That was many years ago. Billy Jean has been able to maintain her beautifully landscaped home over the years. It hasn't always been easy. There have been some months or even years when Billy Jean has barely gotten by. There have been some weeks when the weeds have grown out of control, but Billy Jean has never let it get out of hand. She knows that getting on track and cleaning up the small mess is easier than letting the weeds grow and having to start over from the beginning. Despite the little bumps in the road, Billy Jean has always kept her garden looking as gorgeous as it was when she first cleaned it up. The best part about this story is Billy Jean truly enjoys gardening now and wants to do it.

Billy Jean, you never looked so good!

What am I saying? I am saying that if you do this correctly, you will enjoy it. If you enjoy it, you will want to incorporate it into your lifestyle. It needs to be realistic and sustainable. If Billy Jean disliked gardening, she could never maintain her gardening. If she didn't go out there with an open mind, she would not be able to succeed. I am certain there were days when the bugs were bad. I know there were days where Billy Jean was tired or it was raining. Billy Jean stayed positive, and her attitude radiated through in her actions.

Let's talk about attitude, shall we?

By now, I have already told you that it's not going to be easy. You understand that this will be a grueling process if you allow it to be—*if* you allow it to be. Much like a pregnancy. Being pregnant is not the most wonderful slice of heaven. At times, it sucks. It is also the most amazing, miraculous time that anyone will ever experience. It is agonizing most of the time. In the end, you get the most amazing gift there is.

Much like being pregnant, you don't know what to expect. You can't predict what your body is going to do each day. You just have to deal with it. Like many things in life, your attitude will dictate your actions.

We have all met Betty the Bullfrog. You know, the one who cries and whines about everything. No matter what the scenario is, Betty will find something to complain about. My philosophy has always been to look at the bright side. The glass is always half full. This is the ultimate game changer.

Shit or get off the pot, Betty … No one wants to hear you bitch.

There. I said it. Bullfrogs are bullfrogs because they *want* to be miserable. Their glasses are always half empty. Nothing ever goes their way, and they complain about everything. Bullfrog Betty makes Debbie Downer look like a rock star. Sometimes I catch myself thinking like a bullfrog, and I drop-kick myself to the ground and talk sense into myself. Life is too short.

When you are dieting, you aren't going to love every second. You are going to want to eat cake. You are also going to want to slap people. The worst part is when you don't eat the cake, and you don't lose a pound the next day. This is when you wish you had Bullfrog Betty and Maddie McBoobs side by side with a taser gun.

Word of advice: Anger will get you nowhere. Staying positive will. Keep your eye on the ball. You have to remember that it is the big picture that matters. Much like any goal, you won't understand how fabulous the end result is until you actually see it. It's not tangible until the end. We discussed how it is difficult to grasp abstract concepts earlier in this book. There is nothing I can say that will get you to understand the feeling of feeling good. More importantly, that feeling of feeling good is amplified when you worked so incredibly hard to achieve it. Nothing in the world can top it. No antidepressant. No anxiety med. No drug or substance could make you feel this good—the way you can feel just by treating your body the way it should be treated.

Initially, people who don't understand the positive repercussions of this will be negative. Many of them will complain. Most of them will quit. Those who persevere will cross the horizon of darkness and see the glowing light. As long as you embrace the light and stay positive, you will be comfortable on this side and never cross back. You'll know when you get here.

I can't explain it, but when you cross over, you just know all the people who are part of this club. There's no name for our group. There's no club or association. It's just a metaphysical society that those of us belong to who understand the importance of this lifestyle. It's not something we think about anymore. Once you are here, you don't ever doubt your membership. You know you are never leaving, much like your citizenship.

As a member of this society, we can always tell when there are people who are trying to transition into our group. Often the transition is successful. Many times, it is not, and the foreigner ends up leaving our club only to return again at a later time. Once you are a resident, it is unlikely that you would ever leave. Your mind-set and attitude have been forever changed. You truly love your newly adapted lifestyle. You have no desire to have a cheat meal or eat poorly. A bad eating day is considered a day that you didn't get all of your nutrients in. Exercising makes you feel good. It isn't something you have to force yourself to do. In fact, you have to schedule a rest day in order to give your body a break. It's a great place to be. The greatest place on earth.

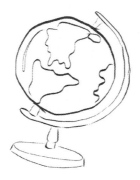

There are no haters here.

Everyone embraces others' successes.

We only look at the facts.

We don't compete with others, only ourselves.

We don't make excuses.

We don't lie to ourselves.

We don't get frustrated.

There are no shortcuts.

There are no bullfrogs.

We don't cheat or cut in line.

Self-forgiveness is a must.

We learn from our mistakes.

Food is our fuel.

We keep it real.

We practice patience.

There are no askholes here.

Praise the positive.

We don't judge.

We love ourselves.

If you have faith in this process, it will bring you good things … just like Santa. The more you believe in the process, the more you will believe in yourself. People can't get very far with any goal when they have a tarnished view of themselves.

Positive thinking brings positive results.

Positive results create positive attitudes that generate positive thoughts.

Positive qualities bring positive characteristics that spiral into positive outlooks.

Positive underlying tones will cultivate positive environmental attributes that will bring positive viewpoints.

Positive perspectives will fabricate positive internal standpoints that could lead to permanent positive mind-sets.

Positive implementation of applications will undergo positive involvement with the exposure of positive participation and insights with positive theoretical and spiritual psyches.

For the love of God, do you get it already?

I'm laughing out loud thinking about you dumbasses reading those last six sentences thinking WTF is she on …

Just trust the damn process, okay?

Don't fuck with it. Just don't.

It will beat you every time.

It has never lost.

It is stronger than you if you allow it to be.

You have to be the alpha and show it who is boss.

Don't let it defeat you.

Once you have established this, you will have no issues. You will have the upper hand.

Things won't bother you.

Your paint brushes won't dry up.

Weight fluctuations won't defeat you.

They are just weeds in your garden than can be clipped away.

It's part of the process.

Weeds will grow.

You will get really good at trimming them.

Don't ever let them get out of control. If you do, then you have to start over. If you have to start over, then you do. I have had to start over so many times I wrote a book about it.

I never formally told my story. If you were paying close attention to the stories throughout the book, they are narratives of pieces of my life. All of them. I am Carissa and Alyky. I am Billy Jean and even Samantha. I have been Avanna, Nikki, and Matteo. I am a master of everything that could go wrong when trying to lose weight.

I was a teacher who gained a ton of weight getting my master's degree. I was called into the teacher's lounge by the Bavarian cream donuts. I tried to get my run in during my lunch hour and isolated myself from the rest of the staff. I had no idea that a mocha had 620 calories. I'm the one with the True Religion imprint on my ass. I have cut in line. I have weighed myself at noon after working out. I've eaten sleeves of cookies and bought more gadgets than I can recall. I have lied to myself. I have used all the excuses. I have skipped breakfast. I have tried detoxes. I have been unrealistic. I have self-sabotaged. I have painted a beautiful mural and scribbled over it with black paint. I've watched the gargoyles party like rock stars while the wrecking ball destroyed all my hard work.

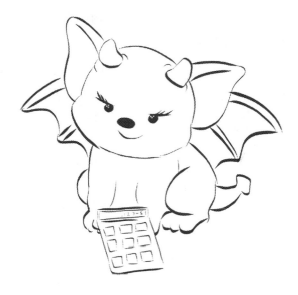

I went out to eat and ordered vodka water and had a strawberry for dessert to find that I didn't do good. I skipped my afternoon snack only to end up eating thousands of calories of carrots and almonds. I have groomed my landscaping to be perfect, only to watch the weeds take over and grow. The weeds still take over from time to time, but I always know what I have to do to keep it managed. I have taken every single mistake and learned from it. I have had to learn to grow and self-reflect. I have learned about the process and over time gained the strength to trust it.

Trust the process. Trust the process. Trust the process. Trust the process. Trust the process.

Trust the process. Trust the process. Trust the process. Trust the process. Trust the process.

I don't have time to cook. I have had to put the frickin' chicken in the oven. I didn't have time to work out; in fact, I didn't even like it. I dreamed of being a runner—just a fantasy I had. I can't tell you how many times I bought running shoes and darted out the door with my ponytail swinging behind me, only to return in disappointment. I had two things on my bucket list back then. One was to run a marathon. The other was to write a book. Both things required a lot more spiritual and mental strength than I ever thought I could possess.

Fifty marathon finishes later I sit here, finishing my first book. The wife of a physically fit PE teacher and mother of four amazing children, and I still have excuses. I still don't have time. I still get tired. I still love long Johns, and I definitely still get crabby. The gargoyles still visit me on occasion … especially at three o'clock. #hiswifeatedonuts

I have learned a lot. I have learned to be patient. I have learned to self-forgive, to be flexible, and to understand there is no set plan. I have learned to love myself. I don't deprive myself, yet I know to keep it real. Realistic, sustainable expectations. I have learned to accept every mistake and make it a lesson. I embrace that. I have learned that this process is a very complicated but rewarding one. It must be trusted in order for it to work.

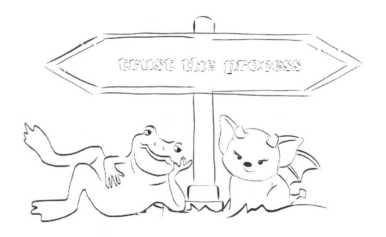

Believe, and you shall receive.

Trust the process ...

Keep fucking going ...

And don't ever stop ...

Printed in the United States
By Bookmasters